Twist Me Pretty
BRAIDS

45 Step-by-Step Tutorials
for Beautiful, Everyday Hairstyles

ABBY SMITH

ULYSSES
PRESS

Published by:
Ulysses Press
P.O. Box 3440
Berkeley, CA 94703
www.ulyssespress.com

ISBN: 978-1-61243-728-6
Library of Congress Control Number: 2017938181

Printed in China

10 9 8 7 6 5

Acquisitions editor: Casie Vogel
Managing editor: Claire Chun
Editor: Shayna Keyles
Proofreader: Renee Rutledge
Design and layout: Malea Clark-Nicholson

Contents

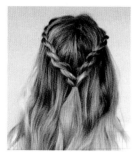

Beach Twists **12**

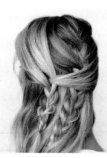

Bohemian Braids **15**

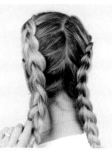

Boxer Braids **18**

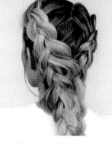

Formal Boxer Braids **21**

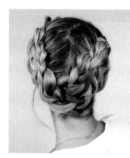

Boxer Halo Braids **22**

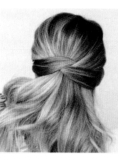

Easy Half Up **24**

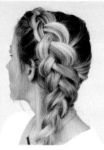

Dutch Side Braid **26**

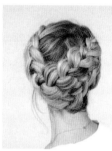

Crown Braid **28**

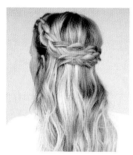

Half Crown Braid **30**

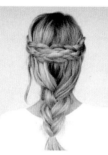

Mixed Crown Braid **33**

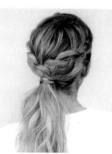

Braided Ponytail **34**

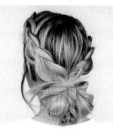

Dutch Braided Bun **36**

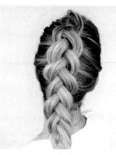

Faux Hawk Braid **39**

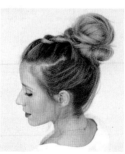

Faux Hawk Bun **41**

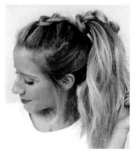

Faux Hawk Ponytail **43**

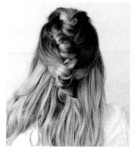

Knotted Faux Hawk with Extensions **47**

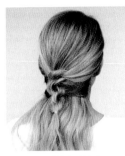

Knotted Half Up **50**

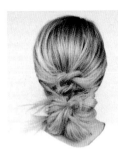

Knotted Updo **53**

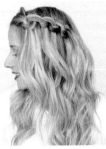

Looped Accent Braid **55**

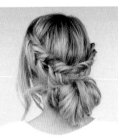

Fishtail Updo **59**

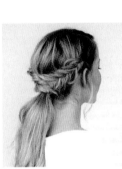

Fishtail Ponytail **61**

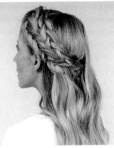

Mixed Braids **62**

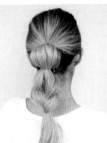

Mixed Ponytail **65**

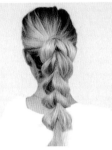

Pull Through Ponytail **67**

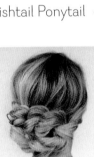

Pull Through Updo **71**

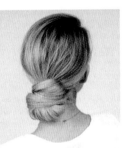

Simple Bun **75**

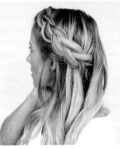

Soft Dutch Braid **77**

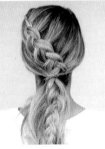

Sideways Dutch Ponytail **79**

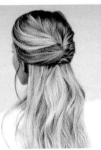

Topsy Tail Half Up **81**

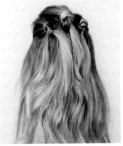

Triple Knots **83**

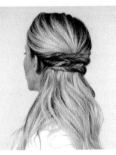

Twisted Crown Braid **86**

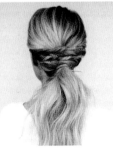

Twisted Crown Ponytail **88**

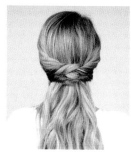

Twisted Half Up **91**

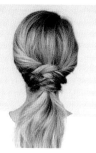

Twisted Half
Ponytail **93**

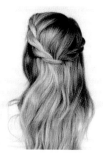

Twisted Crown **95**

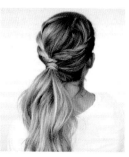

Twisted Ponytail **98**

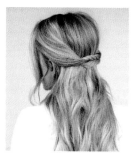

Twisted
Together **101**

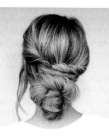

Twisted Together
Bun **103**

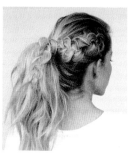

Viking Braid **105**

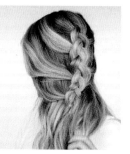

Uneven Center
Braid **108**

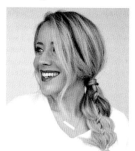

Four-Strand
Braid **111**

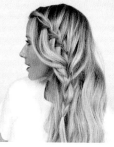

Draped Waterfall
Braid **113**

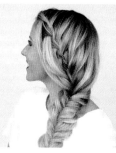

Draped Waterfall
Fishtail Braid **117**

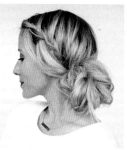

Waterfall Messy
Bun **119**

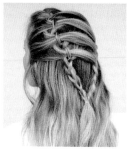

Corset Braid **121**

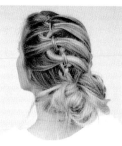

Corset Braid and
Bun **125**

Introduction

WELL, HELLO!

My name is Abby; it's nice to meet you! I'm so happy this book has finally made it into your hands, and I hope it inspires you with fresh new hairstyles every day. My favorite place to keep it is in the bathroom—for those crazy mornings when you're rushed on time and low on inspiration. This book can be a great resource for you when you're in a hurry and need something quick, or you might use it to help you get dolled up for a fancy wedding or holiday party. Whatever your event, I hope your style makes you feel as gorgeous as you are!

This book isn't going to cover everything… I mean c'mon, there's only so much a girl can do in 128 pages! But I do hope these hairstyles inspire you to try something new and to be a little more brave and creative! After all, your hair is one of your best accessories. It's an easy place for you to experiment and express the way you're feeling. I promise, if you spend a few extra minutes each morning to give yourself a little TLC, you'll find a boost in your confidence and attitude toward yourself and others.

A LITTLE BIT ABOUT ME

I'm a self-taught, hair-obsessed blogger and YouTuber with four small kids and a passion for beauty. I'm a firm believer that you can do *anything* you set your mind to. Believe it or not, before I started this journey, I couldn't even French braid my own hair! I didn't know anything about blogging, photography, filming videos, or how the world of social media works. But I've always loved the saying, "Hard work beats talent if talent doesn't work hard." So if you want something, go out there and get it!

You're about to learn a handful of new skills and techniques by reading this book, and I'm sure it'll test your patience at times. But please, don't get discouraged. It'll all be worth it when you finally master those hairstyles and people start complimenting your beautiful braids.

All of these hairstyles can be found on my YouTube channel—just search Twist Me Pretty. If you're struggling with a style, go watch me teach you how to master it in person. You'll find that it's super helpful to have a real voice and real hands show you how it's done. Use this book to help remind you what comes next and to give you inspiration when yours is running low. And remember that when you're having trouble, you can always reach out to me! Find me on my website at twistmepretty.com or on Instagram @twistmepretty.

Let's just be bffs already, mmk?!

BASIC BRAIDS YOU SHOULD KNOW

- **The French Braid**, where the outer strands go OVER the middle. This is your foundational braid. If you can conquer the French braid, the rest will follow!

- **The Dutch Braid**, where the outer strands go UNDER the middle. This braid pops off the head and is perfect for pictures or when you want that gorgeous texture to show.

- **The Fishtail Braid**, where you crisscross strands from two sections to form an intricate-looking braid. This braid is one of the easier styles to master, but it looks incredibly complicated!

- **The Waterfall Braid**, where you drop and replace a section of your French braid. Interestingly enough, it looks just like a waterfall!

We covered these braids in my last book, *The New Braiding Handbook*, so I haven't gone into great detail here, but if you need a reminder, make sure to hit up my basic braids videos.

Pro Tip: Don't watch yourself in the mirror when you're learning these braids. Just say the steps out loud as you go, and remember that it's okay if you don't get it the first time around. Practice makes perfect!

BUILDABLE HAIRSTYLES

I love buildable hairstyles, and you will find several throughout this book. These are styles that build upon each other. For example, a crown braid can be worn as a regular crown braid with curls, or you can build upon it by adding a low bun or a fishtail braid onto the ends. These hairstyles typically elevate somewhat simple, basic styles.

A FEW THINGS YOU'LL NEED

- **Strong bobby pins.** You can never underestimate the power of a strong bobby pin! Ditch the cheap ones and upgrade; it'll save your hairstyling life. I use MetaGrip Premium Bobby Pins, but just make sure you're buying pins that pinch closed, won't bend when you're trying to open them, and have a soft tip so you don't damage your hair!

- **A 1-inch curling wand.** I wrapped my hair around a 1-inch curling wand to get the waves you see in the photos in this book. I love the 1-inch size because it holds the curl for several days and they just get more and more relaxed as time goes on.

Pro Tip: If you want your curls loose and wavy, pull the curled section immediately after releasing it from the wand. Doing this will release some of the bounce in the curl.

- **Stretchy clear elastics.** I like my clear elastics to stretch easily. I find it's a little bit softer on my hair.

- **A seam ripper.** Say what?! It's a sewing tool used to help rip unwanted seams. I like to use it to help cut out clear elastics! It's great because it's so precise and will save your hair a lot of damage. You can find them in the craft or sewing section at most stores.

- **Two mirrors.** It's extremely helpful to have a mirror in front of you *and* a mirror behind you so that you can see what you're doing while you're doing it. Trust me, it will make your life so much easier!

- **Great hair products**. It's very important to invest in the products you're using on your hair! Especially if you're spending money to color it every couple of months. The products I'm loving are constantly evolving, so make sure to find me on my blog at twistmepretty.com for up-to-date favs.

- **Hair extensions.** These are great for those pin-worthy hairstyles! If you feel like playing around with a little extra thickness or length, my girl Lacy from Laced Hair Extensions has the best clip-ins. I think extensions are so fun to have when you're styling hair. They make your braids bigger, your curls prettier, and it's fun to have all that extra hair to play with.

Well, are you ready to get started? I sure am! If you have any questions, if you're struggling at all, come find me! And do you know what I'd *love*? If you'd share your creations with me—I'm dying to see them! Use the hashtag #twistmepretty so I can search all your beautiful styles and we can all be inspired by your creativity.

Alright, alright, enough already. Turn the page!

The Braids

BEACH TWISTS

This is one of my favorite hairstyles to wear in the summer or to the beach because it keeps my hair out of my face, and if you end up on a boat, it looks way cute in a ponytail, too!

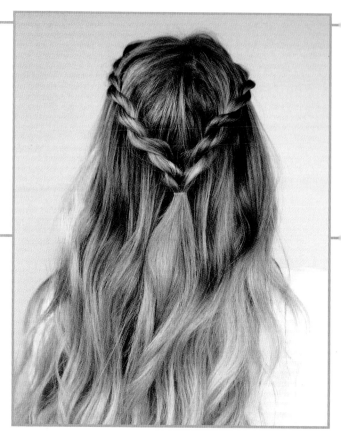

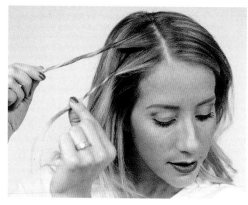

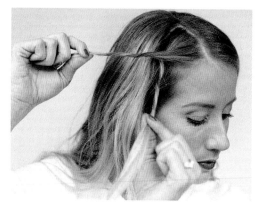

1. Give yourself a slightly centered part. Take a small triangle-shaped section from one side and split it in two. Twist both sections toward your face.

2. Twist the two sections together, twisting away from your face.

Twist Me Pretty Braids

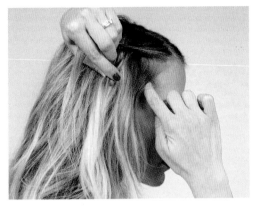

3. Add in a new section to the bottom piece.

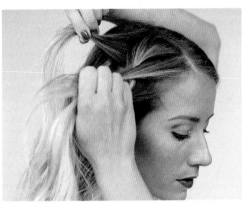

4. Add in a new section to the top piece.

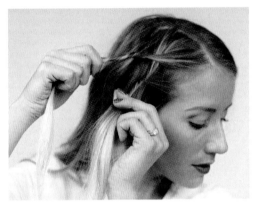

5. Twist each section toward your face, like in step 1.

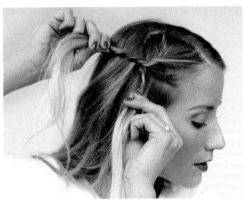

6. Twist the two sections together, twisting away from your face.

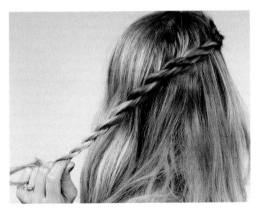

7. Repeat steps 3 through 6 until you reach the back of your head. When you reach the back, do a regular twist all the way down.

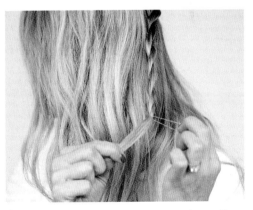

8. Secure with an elastic band or clip.

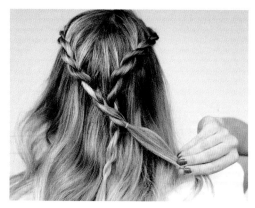

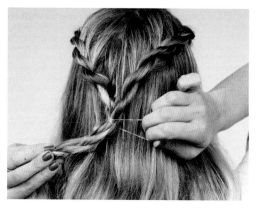

9. Repeat steps 1 through 8 on the other side of your head.

10. Secure the sections together near the crown with a clear elastic band.

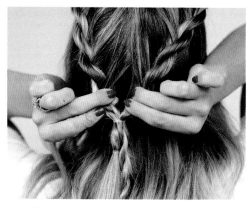

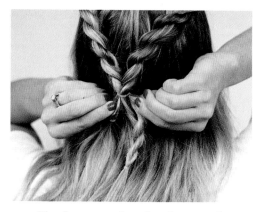

11. Right above the elastic, make a little hole, and flip the hair through.

12. Cinch up on the elastic to make sure it's nice and tight, and then remove the elastics at the bottom of the individual twists.

Pro Tip:

If you put some pomade or gel on your fingers before you start your twist, it'll keep all those pesky flyaways down. And to give the curls some extra texture, spray with a texturizing spray or dry shampoo!

BOHEMIAN BRAIDS

This is such a beautiful down style, something that's casual enough to go run errands in but fancy enough for a date night or school dance!

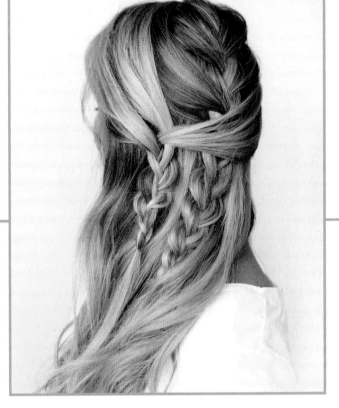

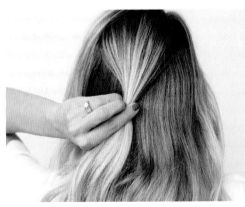

1. Gather a section of hair from the back. Leave two sections of hair, one on each side, near the front of your face for the second braid.

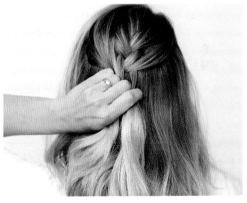

2. Split the section in the back into three sections and start a basic French braid. Remember, in a French braid, the outer strands go over the middle.

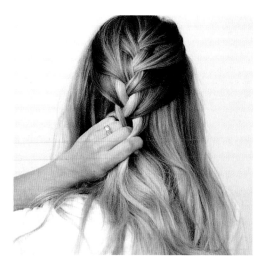

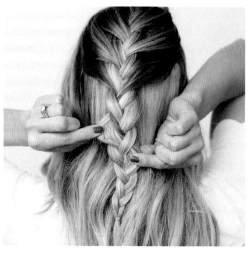

3. When you get about four or five stitches down, quit French braiding and finish it off with a regular three-strand braid all the way down.

4. Secure with a clear elastic and fluff out the braid so it looks more full and voluminous.

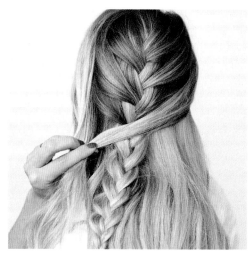

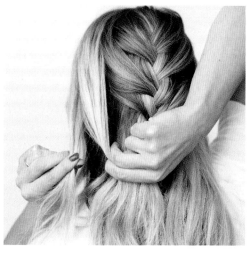

5. Take the two sections of hair from the front of your face. Cross one section over the braid. The other should sit right next to the braid.

6. Split the section that's next to the braid into two sections.

Twist Me Pretty Braids

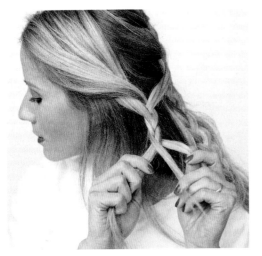

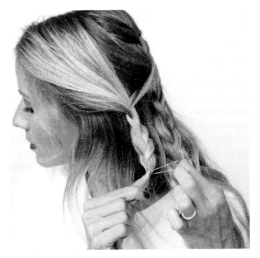

7. Now that you have three sections, go ahead and do a three-strand braid all the way down.

8. Secure with a clear elastic and then spread apart the braid to make it look more full.

BOXER BRAIDS

This is one of the trendiest hairstyles right now—these boxer braids will not disappoint! They'll amp up any workout or make you look super chic and flirty when heading to class or running errands. I also love that there are a million ways to alter the boxer braid, so one style gives you many different looks.

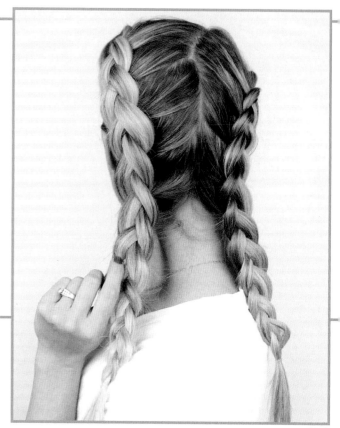

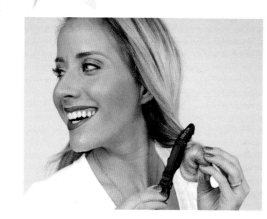

1. Split the hair in half and secure one side with a clip.

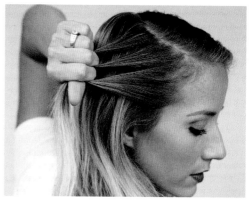

2. Take a small section of hair from the front and divide it into three equal sections. Start your Dutch braid. Remember, in a Dutch braid, the outer strands go under the middle section.

Twist Me Pretty Braids

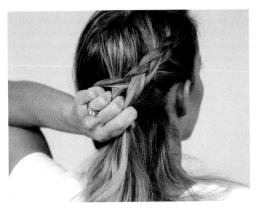

3. Continue braiding all the way down, adding in new sections of hair as you go.

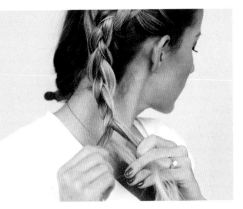

4. When you get to the nape of your neck, finish braiding all the way to the end, and tie off with a clear elastic.

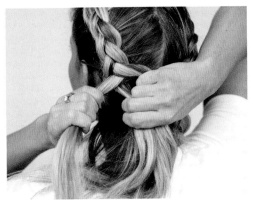

5. Repeat steps 2 through 4 on the other side.

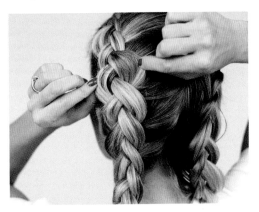

6. Spread apart the braids by gently tugging on the sections of hair. This will open up the braids and make them look more full and voluminous.

Pro Tip:

If you're wearing extensions, use your single wefts for this hairstyle. Put them in near the beginning of the braid and as you spread it apart at the end, you'll cover any wefts that are still visible.

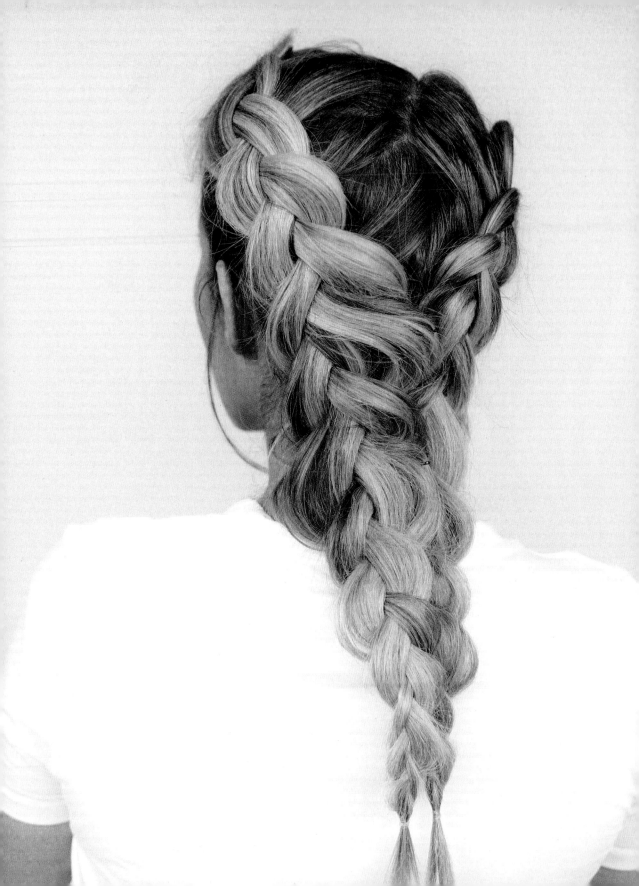

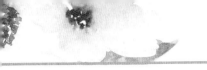

FORMAL BOXER BRAIDS

This is such an elegant braid and a perfect example of a buildable hairstyle. You start with the boxer braids and elevate it into this beautiful style!

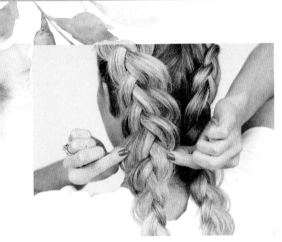

1. Start with the Boxer Braids (page 18). Pull apart the braids to make them look extra thick.

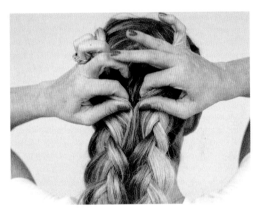

2. Pull the braids close together near the crown of the head.

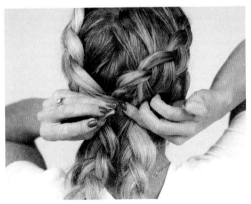

3. Folding one braid over the other, take a bobby pin, snag a small section of hair with it, and then push the bobby pin in toward the bottom braid.

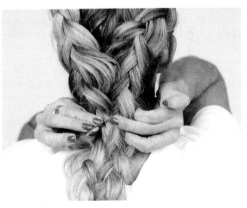

4. Hold the braids together near the nape of the neck and secure them with another bobby pin.

BOXER HALO BRAIDS

This hairstyle is great for those of you with medium-length hair! If you have the length, go ahead and wrap your Dutch braid all the way around and secure on the opposite side with bobby pins.

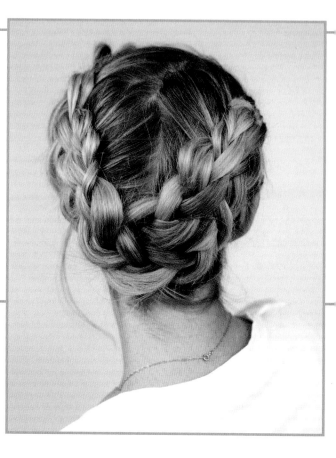

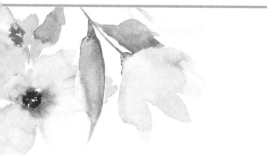

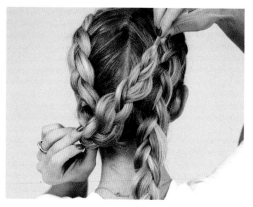

1. Start with Boxer Braids (page 18). Take the tail of one of the braids and fold it up toward the top of the other braid.

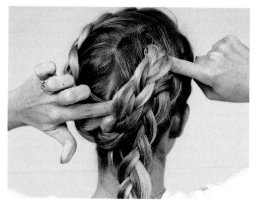

2. Curl the braid over your finger, if the braid is long enough.

Twist Me Pretty Braids

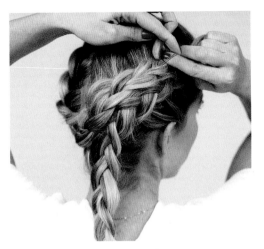

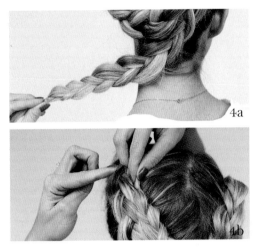

4a

4b

3. Secure with bobby pins.

4. Take the second braid and wrap it over the first. Secure in place with bobby pins just like you did with the first.

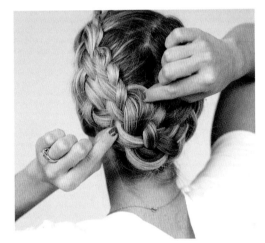

5. Spread apart the braids to make them look extra thick and full.

Pro Tip:

If your hair is clean, you might find it's too slippery. Use some dry shampoo or texturizing spray so the hair has better grip!

EASY HALF UP

This hairstyle is so simple, yet looks so fancy! If you're in a hurry but need to make an impression, this is the hairstyle to pick.

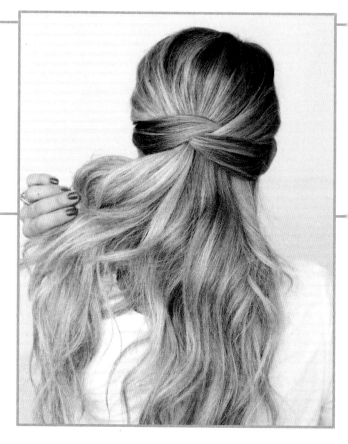

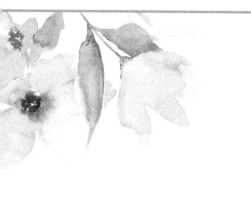

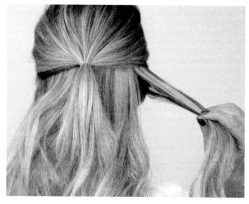

1. Pull the hair half up and secure with a clear elastic. Then, take a small section near the right ear.

2. Create a hole on the left side with your index finger and thumb, then pull the section through.

Twist Me Pretty Braids

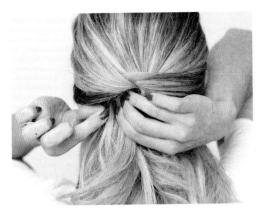

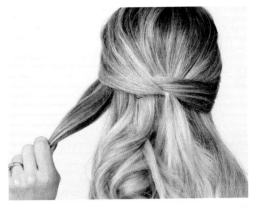

3. Secure with a bobby pin.

4. Gather another section near the left ear.

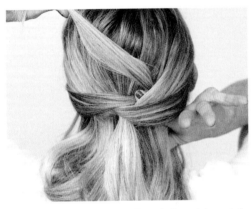

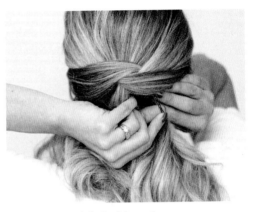

5. Create a hole on the right side with your index finger and thumb, and pull the section through.

6. Secure with bobby pins.

Pro Tip:

Make sure you are using strong bobby pins. If your bobby pins are folding in on themselves or they're not holding up the hair, invest in some stronger pins! I also like to match the color of bobby pins to my hair color so that they're not as noticeable.

DUTCH SIDE BRAID

This is one of those fabulous braids that's perfect for chasing the kids around all day, or it can be something you'd wear to a black tie event. It's completely versatile, perfect to wear on dirty hair, easy to style, and absolutely stunning. The end.

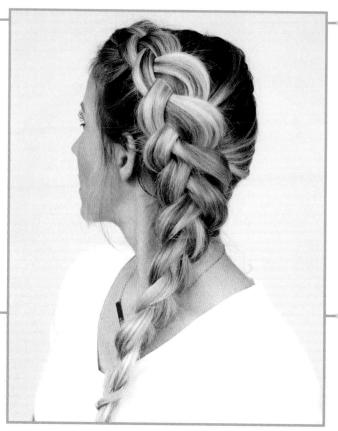

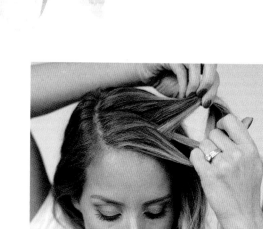

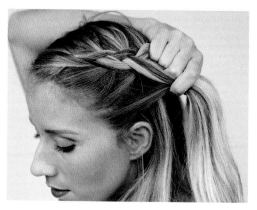

1. Part your hair on the side, then take a large section near the part. Divide it into three sections and braid the outer strands under the middle.

2. Add in new sections of hair on each side and continue Dutch braiding.

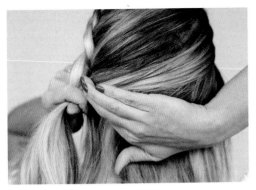

3. Keep the braid close to the front of the head, and continue pulling in hair from the other side. I take fairly large sections from the other side.

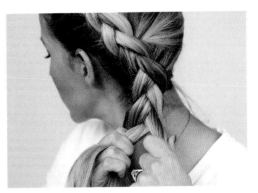

4. When you get to the nape of your neck, start a regular three-strand braid, and braid it all the way down.

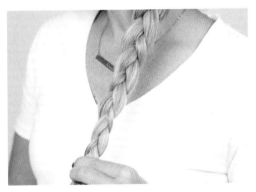

5. Tie it off with a clear elastic.

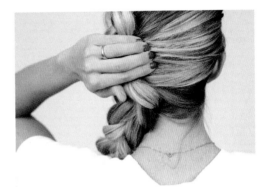

6. Sweep the hair tight into the seam of the braid.

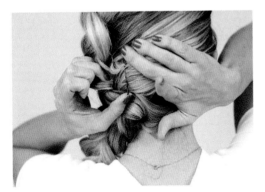

7. Secure the style with bobby pins. Once the rest of the hair feels secure, go ahead and massage the braid, tugging on the sections to make it look extra full and voluminous.

Pro Tip:

Put some mousse or pomade in your fingers while braiding. This will give the braid a nice texture and also help shorter pieces to stay tucked in. If you want to wear extensions, clip them in off-center, toward the side of the braid.

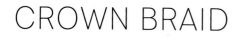

CROWN BRAID

This style is definitely a fav! It works best on medium-length hair because the sections fit together perfectly. The Dutch braids give this hairstyle a lot of great texture and make it a very forgiving style.

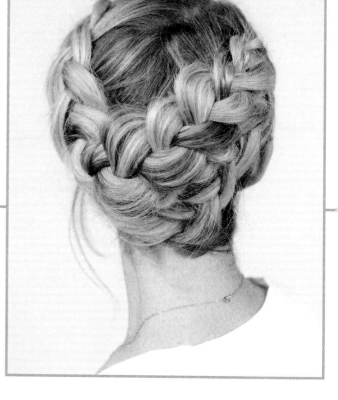

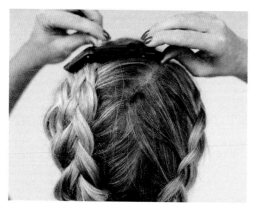

1. Start with Boxer Braids (page 18). Pull one of the braids up into a clip.

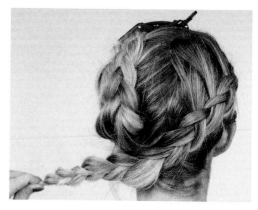

2. Pull the other braid all the way out, across the back of the head.

Twist Me Pretty Braids

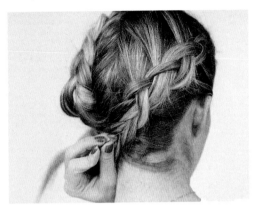

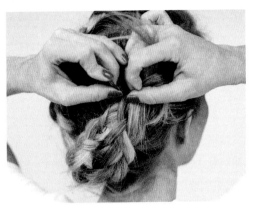

3. Pin it in place at the nape of your neck with bobby pins.

4. Fold the braid back up so that its tail is parallel to the root. Then, tuck the tails underneath the root and secure with bobby pins.

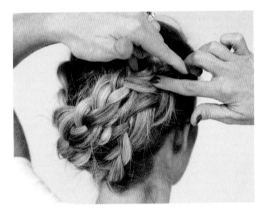

5. Release the other braid from the clip and lay it over the pinned braid. Hide any of the tails underneath the braid and secure with bobby pins.

Pro Tip:

Spread the braids to hide any pins and to make the braids look more voluminous! To keep any flyaways from showing, put some hairspray, pomade, or gel onto your fingertips while styling.

HALF CROWN BRAID

This braid is a great base to many hairstyles! You could put the ends into a regular three-strand braid, a fishtail, a messy bun, a ponytail, and the list goes on and on. It keeps the hair out of the face and is such an easy hairstyle to pull off.

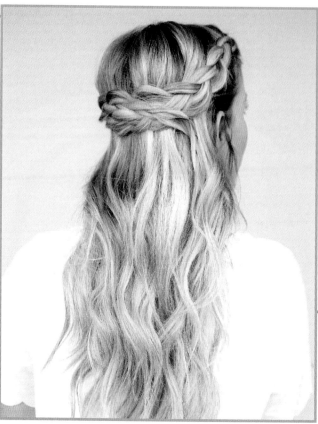

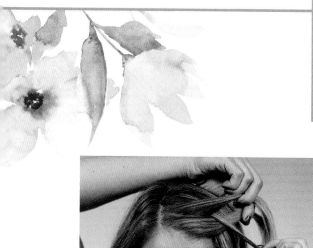

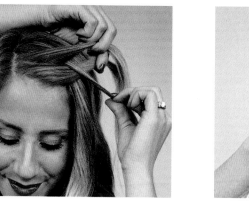

1. Part the hair. On one side, gather a section of hair near the front, divide it into three sections, and braid the outer strands under the middle piece.

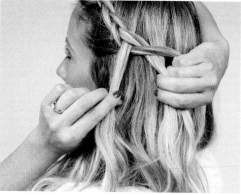

2. Continue Dutch braiding until you reach the ear.

Twist Me Pretty Braids

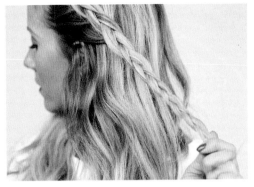

3. Finish off with a three-strand braid.

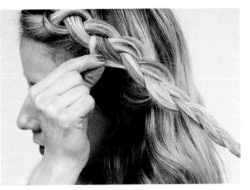

4. Pull apart the braid to make it more fluffy and voluminous.

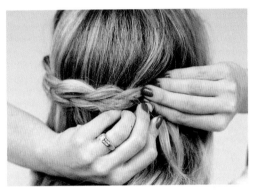

5. Drape it across the crown and secure with a bobby pin.

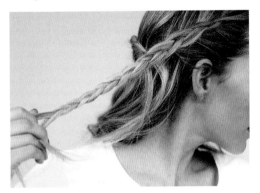

6. Repeat steps 1 through 4 on the other side.

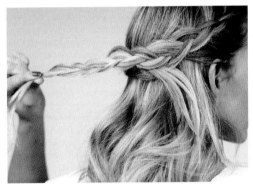

7. Drape the new braid over the first braid.

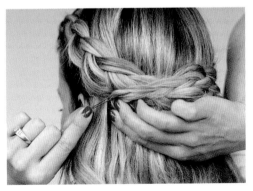

8. Secure with bobby pins.

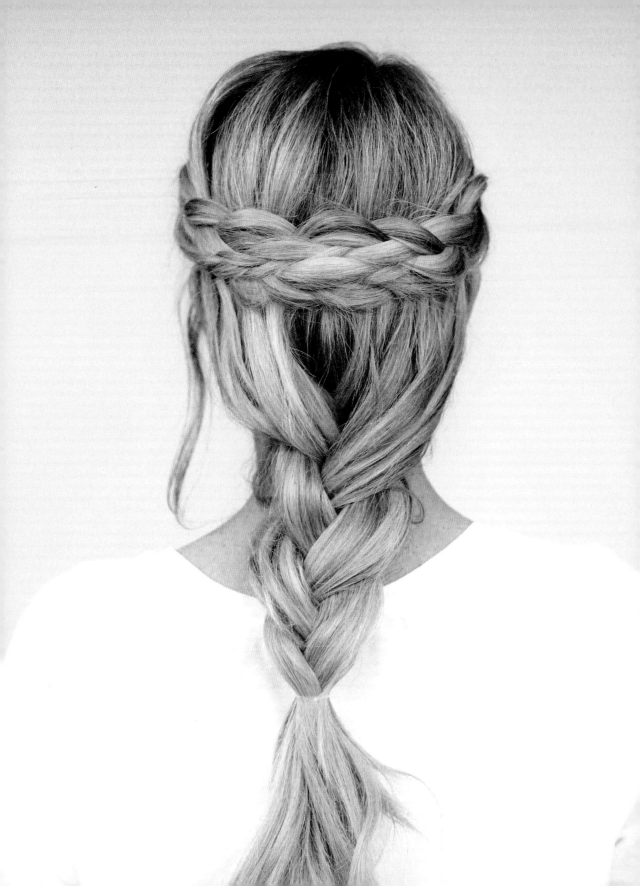

MIXED CROWN BRAID

Some of my favorite hairstyles include simple, mixed braids. Get creative when styling your hair and try to think outside of the box. Combining braids, mixing styles, and putting your own creative touch on your hairstyles is what makes you YOU! I'm choosing to do a regular three-strand braid below, but a fishtail or rope twist would be just as cute!

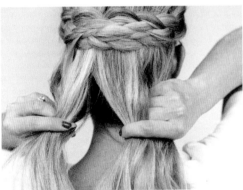

1. Start with the Half Crown Braid (page 30). Separate the remaining hair into three sections.

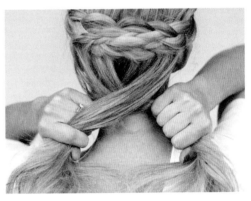

2. Braid all the way down to the ends.

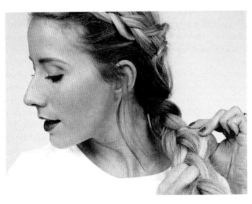

3. Tug on the strands to make the braid more full and voluminous.

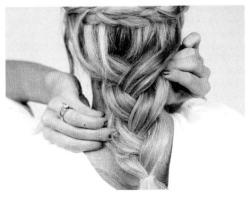

4. Tie off with a clear elastic.

BRAIDED PONYTAIL

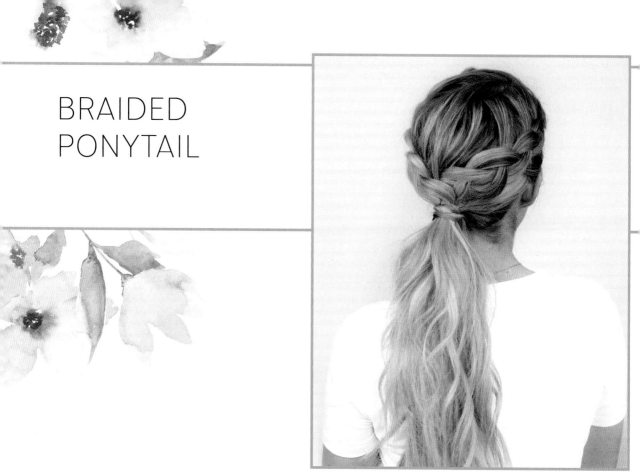

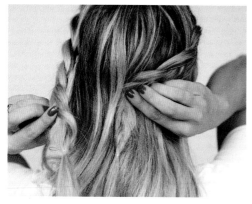

1. Make a Dutch braid on each side of the head and tie them off with a clear elastic.

Pull one braid to the center of the back of your head and hold it down with your index finger.

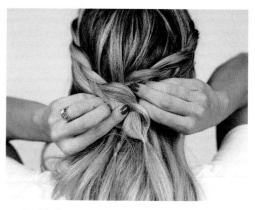

2. Pull the second braid over the first.

Twist Me Pretty Braids

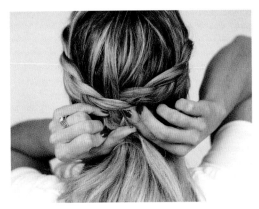

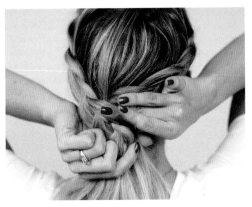

3. Secure both braids with a bobby pin.

4. Take a clear elastic or hair tie and secure the hair, including the braids, into a ponytail.

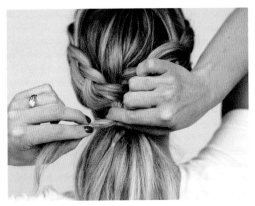

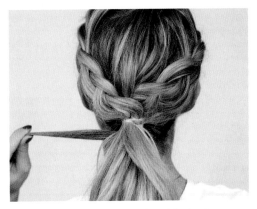

5. Remove the two elastics holding the braids in place.

6. Take a small section of hair from underneath the ponytail.

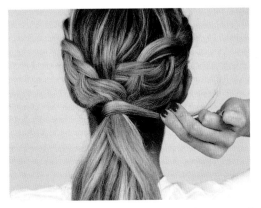

7. Wrap it around the clear elastic and secure with either a bobby pin, or by using another clear elastic.

Pro Tip:

When you're pinning the braids together, make sure you're snagging just enough hair to hold the braids together and that the flat part of your bobby pin is on top. I like to pin just the outside layer of hair because it will hold what's behind it in place. And to hide the pin, just pull apart the braid and it'll disappear!

DUTCH BRAIDED BUN

This is literally my go-to hairstyle. It keeps my hair out of my face while chasing around my kids, it disguises my hair when it's extra dirty, and of course, it's so dang cute!

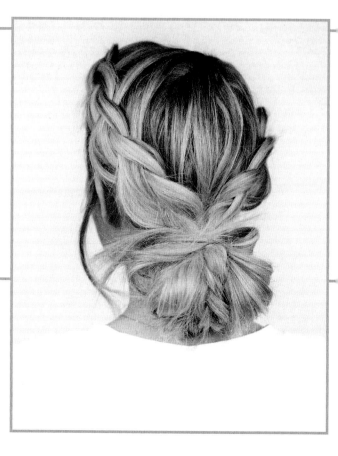

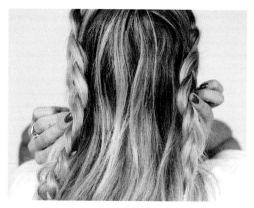

1. Make a Dutch braid on each side of the head and tie them off with a clear elastic.

Pull all the hair back near the nape of your neck.

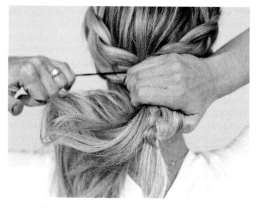

2. Take an elastic and start pulling the hair through.

Twist Me Pretty Braids

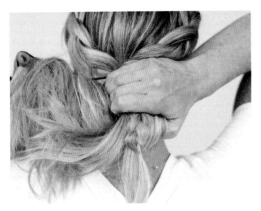

3. When you have a few inches of hair left, twist the elastic.

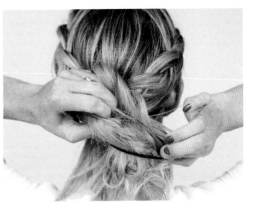

4. Grab the bun with the hand the elastic is on and with your other hand, pull the elastic over the bun.

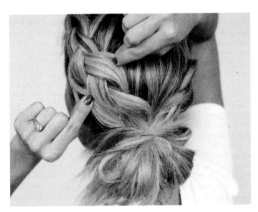

5. Cinch up on the bun to tighten and secure any pieces that popped out with bobby pins. Spread apart the braid to make it look more full and voluminous.

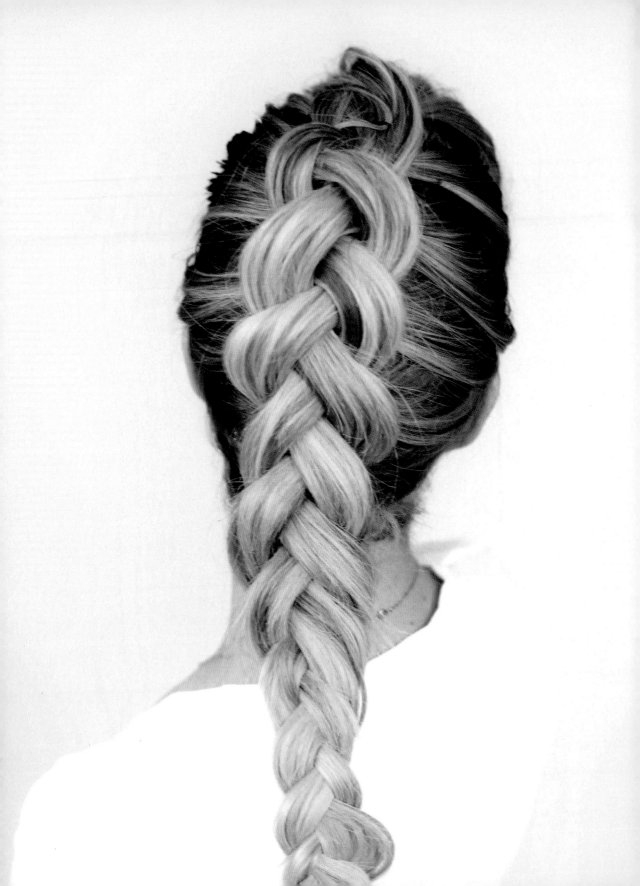

FAUX HAWK BRAID

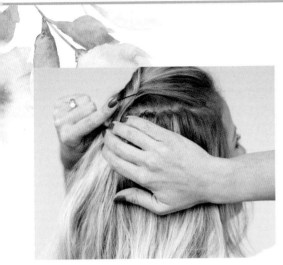

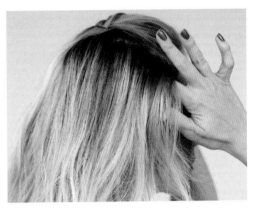

1. Pin back the front section of hair. I like to use this section to give the style more volume.

2. Starting at your temples, gather two sections of hair, one from each side.

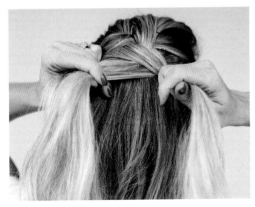

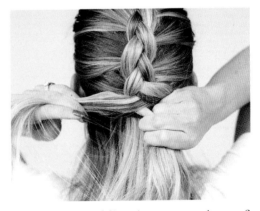

3. Using the tail of your pinned-back section to make your middle section, start your Dutch braid. Remember, you're placing the outer sections underneath the middle section.

4. Continue adding in new sections of hair on each side as you braid down.

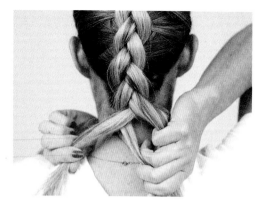

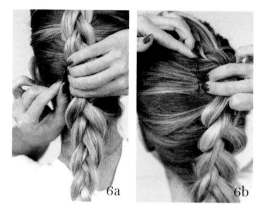

6a

6b

5. When you reach the nape of your neck, finish with a regular three-strand braid, and secure with a clear elastic.

6. Take bobby pins and secure the hair right underneath the Dutch braid. This will help keep those sides nice and tight when you go to fluff out the braid.

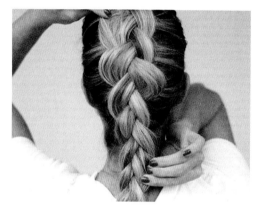

7. Now stretch out your Dutch braid. This will make the braid look extra full, and it will also help hide those bobby pins!

Pro Tip:

To make this braid even edgier, slick back the hair that's coming into the braid by using a comb and some hairspray. Also, pairing it with a bold lip and leather jacket should do the trick!

FAUX HAWK BUN

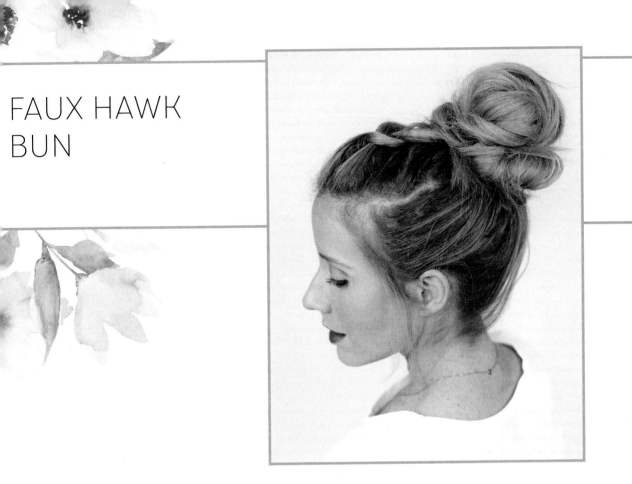

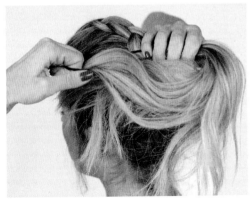

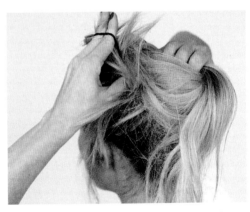

1. Start with steps 1 through 4 of the Faux Hawk Braid (page 39). Pull your hair up into a ponytail, and hold it with the same hand your elastic is on. Using your other hand, pull the elastic over the hair.

2. Leaving just a few inches of ends out, twist the elastic one time.

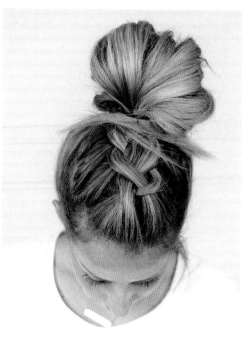

4. Now, all you need to do is cinch up on the bun! By that, I mean find the base of the bun and tighten it by pulling the hair in opposite directions. Then, just tuck any ends that fell out back into the elastic, or use bobby pins to get the shape you want.

Pro Tip:

If your roots are looking a little greasy, use some dry shampoo! This hairstyle is a great second-day hairstyle and styles well on dirty hair.

3. Grab the bun with the hand the elastic is on. Use your other hand to pull the elastic over the bun.

Twist Me Pretty Braids

FAUX HAWK
PONYTAIL

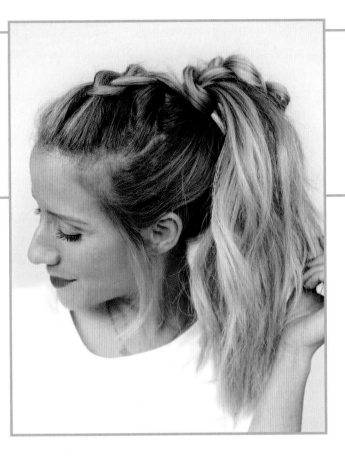

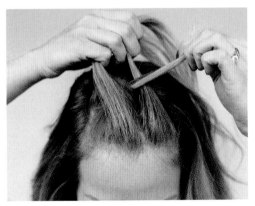

1. Take a section of hair from the front and split it into three. Start your Dutch braid by braiding the outer sections under the middle.

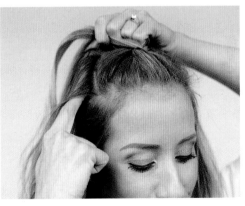

2. Add in new sections of hair on each side.

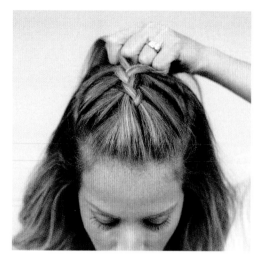

3. Continue braiding to the back.

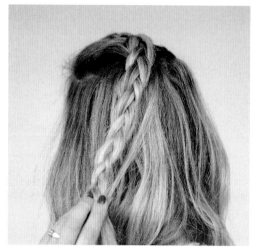

4. Finish the braid off with a regular three-strand braid and secure with a clear elastic.

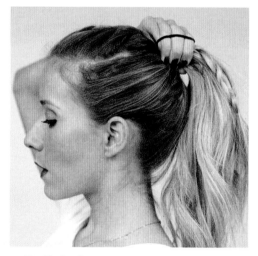

5. Pull the hair up into a ponytail.

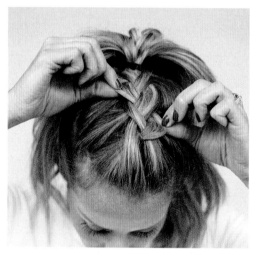

6. Pull apart the braid to make it look more full.

Twist Me Pretty Braids

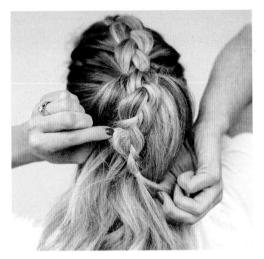

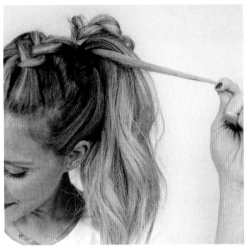

7. If you want, you can stretch the braid all the way down. Or, you can remove the elastic at the bottom of the braid so the braid ends where the ponytail starts.

8. Take a small section of hair from underneath the ponytail and wrap it around the elastic band. Then, secure the piece with either a clear elastic band or with a bobby pin.

Pro Tip:

If your hair is clean when styling this braid, use some texturizing spray or dry shampoo to give the hair a little bit of grip!

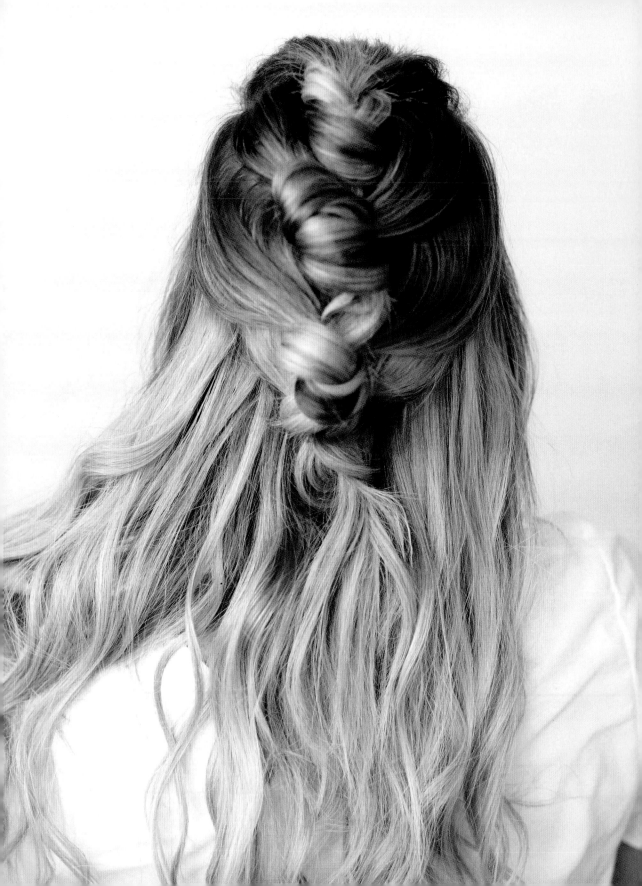

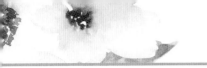

KNOTTED FAUX HAWK WITH EXTENSIONS

This is such a fun hairstyle when you're looking for something a little glam, maybe even edgy. Style it without extensions, though, and you've got yourself a fun everyday 'do!

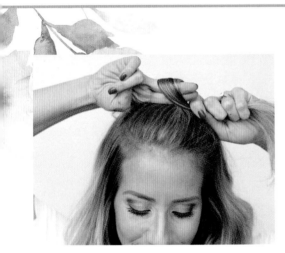

1. Pull back a section of hair from the front of your head. Put two fingers on top of the hair, right before the tail, then bring the tail forward and wrap it over the fingers.

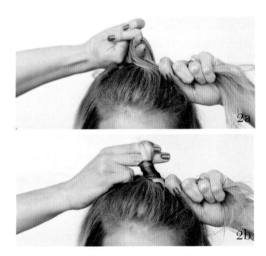

2. Twist your fingers 360 degrees, creating a loop of hair.

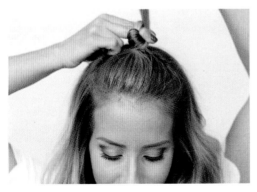

3. Put the tail in between your fingers and pull the tail through the loop of hair. You've just made your first knot!

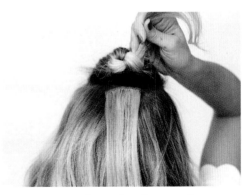

4. Add a single weft of extensions underneath the first knot.

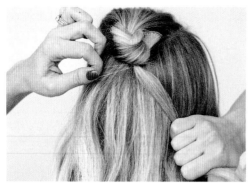

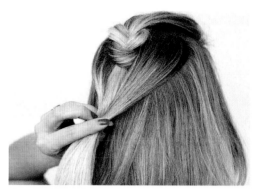

5. Combine the extensions with the tail from the knot and tie them together with a clear elastic. Pull apart the knot just enough to hide the weft and secure as needed with a bobby pin or two.

6. Gather another section of hair right below the knot.

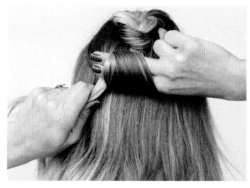

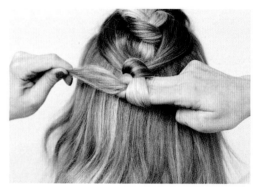

7. Wrap the hair over the fingers.

8. Twist the fingers around and pull the tail through.

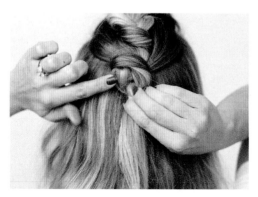

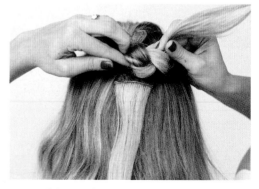

9. Push bobby pins into the knot, crisscrossing if necessary, to secure.

10. Add another single weft extension under the knot.

Twist Me Pretty Braids

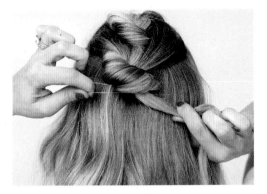 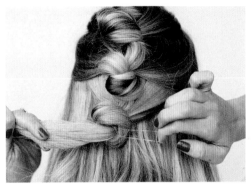

11. Combine the knot and the extensions using a clear elastic.

Continue steps 7 through 11 until you have four or five knots.

12. On the last knot, refrain from adding new hair into the hairstyle and just tie another knot into the tail. Use bobby pins as needed to keep the knots from slipping out.

Pro Tip:

Use hairspray or pomade on your fingers as you knot each section. This will keep the knots smooth and flyaway-free!

KNOTTED HALF UP

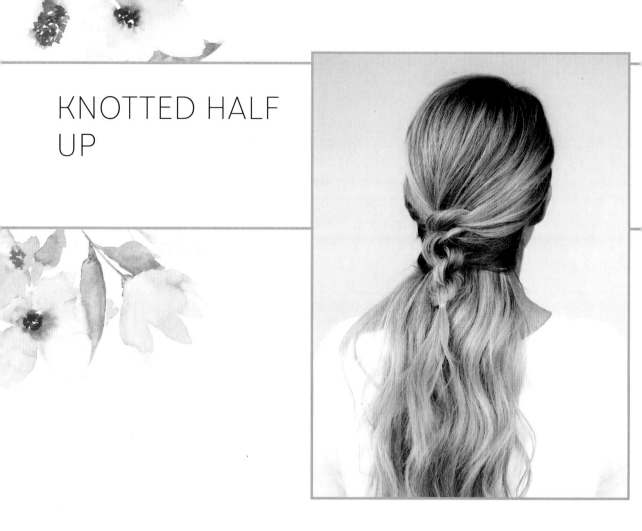

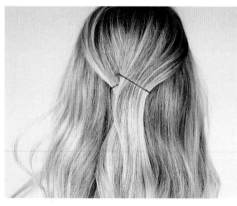

1. Pull a section of hair back and secure it with crisscrossing bobby pins.

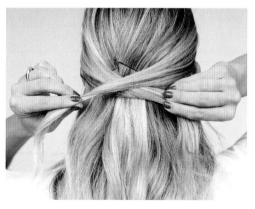

2. Gather two sections of hair near the front of the head, one on each side, and cross them over each other in the back.

Twist Me Pretty Braids

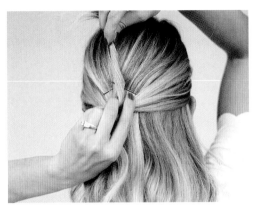

3. If the right section is crossed over the left, pull the left section up (or vice versa).

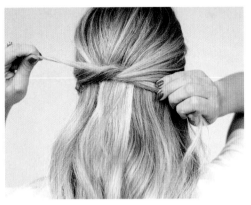

4. Push the left section through the hole between strands to make your first knot.

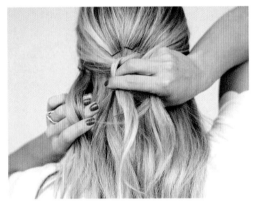

5. Holding the tails, gather a new section of hair on the left side.

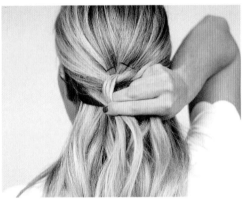

6. Combine the new section with the left strand.

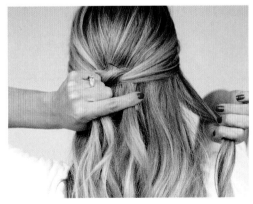

7. Gather a new section of hair on the right side, combine it with the right strand, and make another knot.

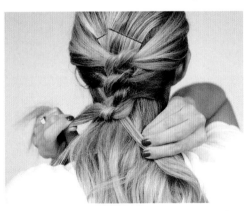

8. Repeat these steps until you reach the nape of your neck.

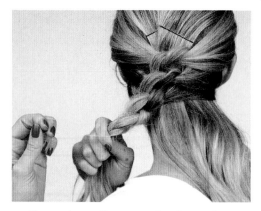

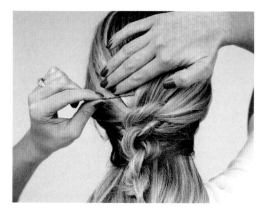

9. Knot the tails a couple times down and secure with a clear elastic.

10. Remove the bobby pins from step 1.

Pro Tip:

If you have really thick hair, try sliding a bobby pin into each knot to keep the knots secure. And if you have really fine hair, make sure to use a texturizing spray or dry shampoo to roughen up the hair before starting your knots!

KNOTTED UPDO

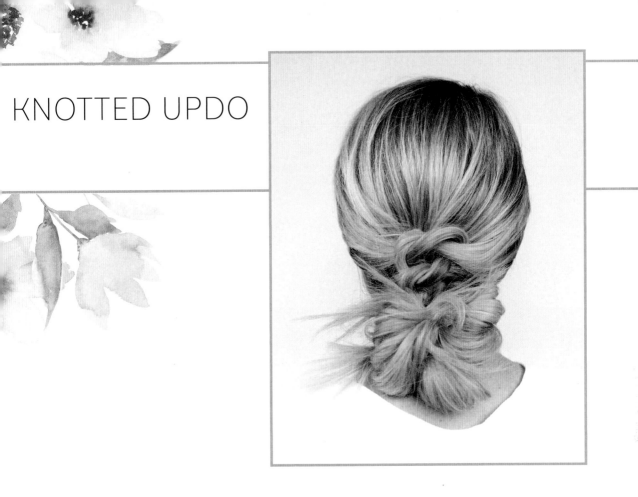

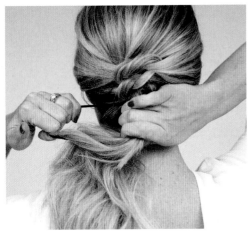

1. Start the Knotted Half Up hairstyle (page 50). Pull the hair into a low ponytail.

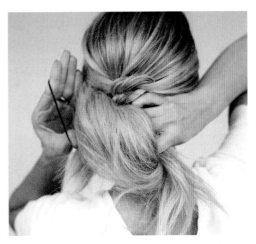

2. Before the ends fall out, twist the elastic one time.

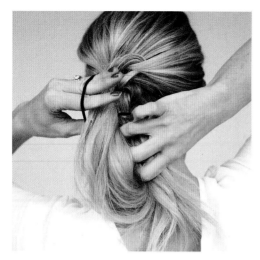 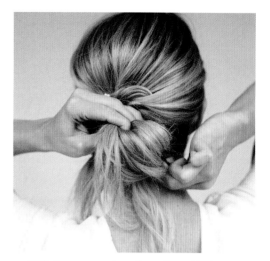

3. Grab the bun with the same hand the elastic is on.

4. With your other hand, pull the elastic over the bun.

5. Cinch up on the bun and secure as needed with bobby pins.

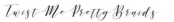

LOOPED ACCENT BRAID

This Looped Accent Braid is such a great style to mix with other braids! It looks so cute thrown up in a messy bun, a side braid, or looped all the way around like a crown braid. Get creative with all the different ways you can wear it!

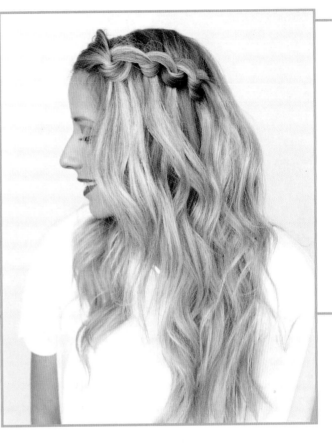

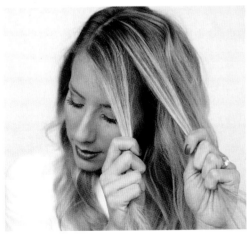

1. Take a section from the heavier side of the part and split it in two.

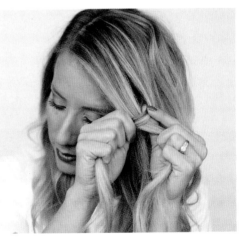

2. Cross the back section over the front section, making sure to leave a hole above where the two sections cross.

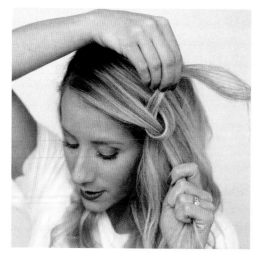

3. Reach under the hole and pull the back section of hair up and through.

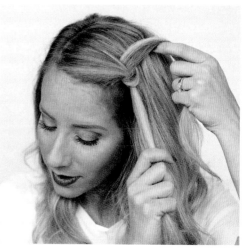

4. Pull gently on both tails, cinching the loop closer up to the part.

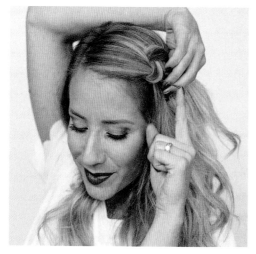

5. Secure the loop by bobby pinning the strand that's hanging straight down.

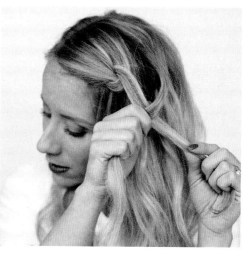

6. Take the top strand from the loop and gather a new section of hair from behind. Cross the back section over the front section.

Twist Me Pretty Braids

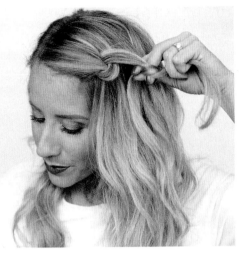

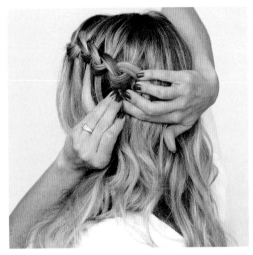

7. Reach under the hole and pull the back section of hair up and through. Secure with a bobby pin, then continue looping sections until you get to the end.

8. When you've looped as far back as you want, secure the ends by adding one bobby pin to the strand that's hanging down.

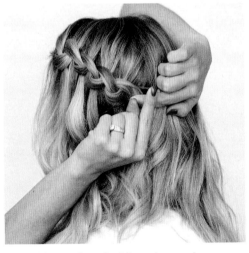

Pro Tip:

Put some pomade or styling mousse in your fingers to help avoid any flyaways! Also, if you start with dirty hair or apply texturizing spray, the bobby pins will hold the loops better!

9. Add another bobby pin to the strand on top.

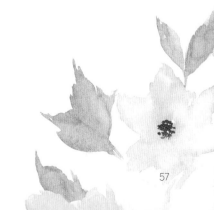

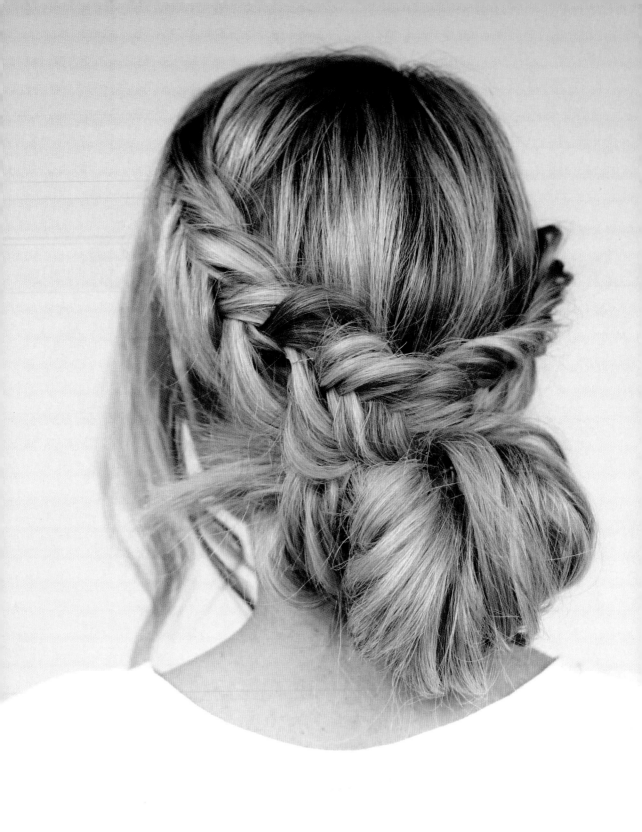

FISHTAIL UPDO

This is one of my favorite updos because it looks so fancy and difficult, but the steps are actually pretty straightforward and easy to follow! Before trying this hairstyle, make sure you are familiar with how to French fishtail braid!

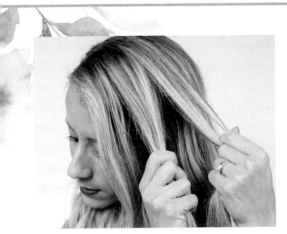

1. Leaving out a section of bangs, gather a small section of hair on one side of your head and split it into two sections.

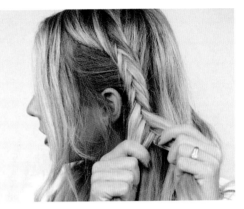

2. Begin your fishtail braid. I like mine to start near the temple. Braid all the way down.

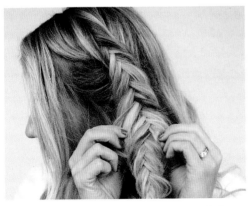

3. Secure with a clear elastic and then flatten the braid by spreading out and tugging on the sections.

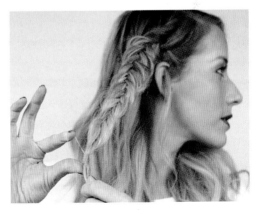

4. Repeat on the other side.

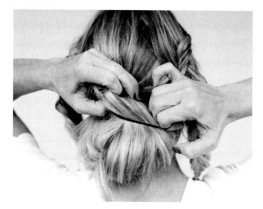

5. Leaving out the two fishtail braids, pull the hair up into a messy bun. Before the ends fall out of a ponytail, twist the elastic band and wrap the elastic over the bun, pulling it with your opposite hand.

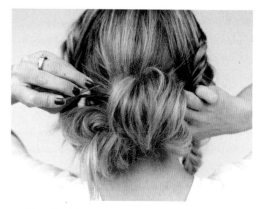

6. Use bobby pins to lift and secure the bun.

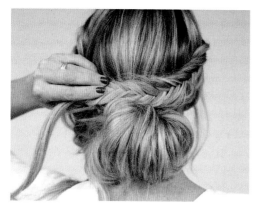

7. Drape one of the fishtail braids over the top of the bun and secure with bobby pins.

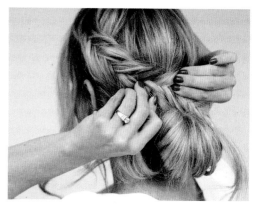

8. Drape the other fishtail braid over the first braid and secure in place with bobby pins.

Pro Tip:

If you want the bun to be extra full, put some extensions in before putting the hair up into a bun.

FISHTAIL PONYTAIL

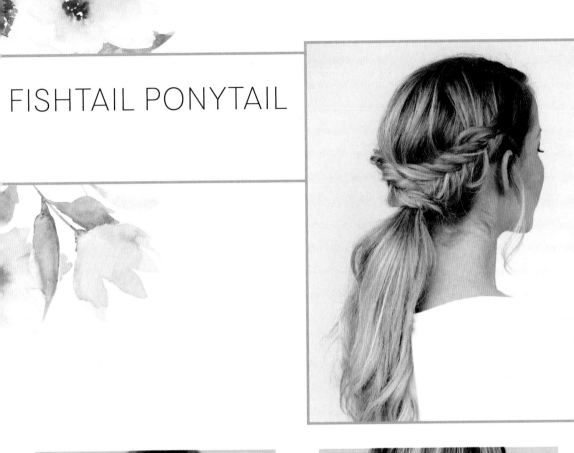

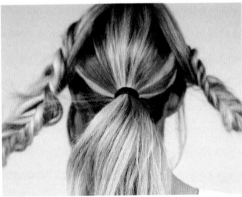

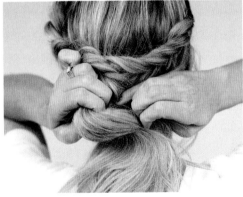

1. Start with steps 1 through 4 of the Fishtail Updo (page 59). Pull your hair up into a ponytail, leaving out the fishtail braids.

2. Drape one fishtail over the ponytail and then drape the other fishtail over the first braid.

3. Wrap the tails of the braids underneath the ponytail and secure by wrapping a clear elastic around the braids and ponytail.

MIXED BRAIDS

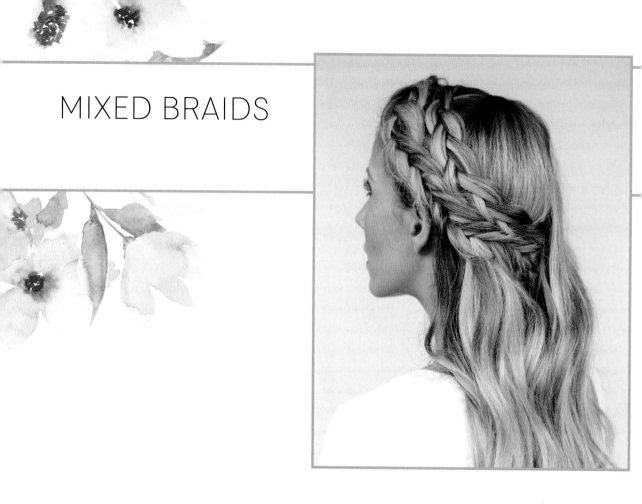

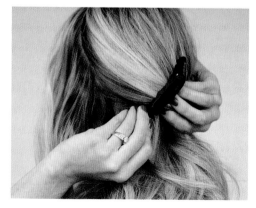

1. On the heavier side of your part, gather a 2-inch section of hair and secure the rest of the hair back with a clip.

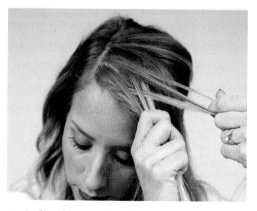

2. Split the section in two and begin your French fishtail braid. For a reminder on how to do this braid, find the tutorial at twistmepretty.com!

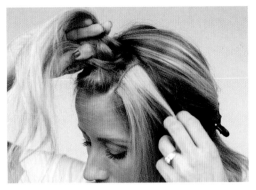

3. If needed, clip in single weft extensions to add volume and thickness to the braid.

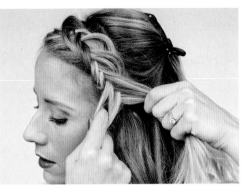

4. Continue French fishtailing all the way down to the ear and then begin a regular fishtail braid.

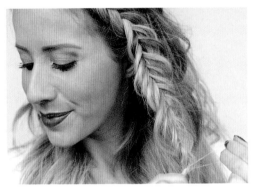

5. When you reach the ends, spread out the braid to make it look full and voluminous, and tie it off with a clear elastic.

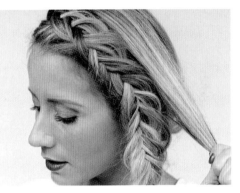

6. Take out another 2-inch section from the clip.

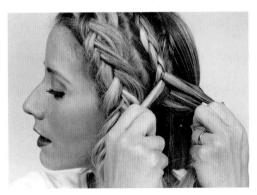

7. Dutch braid all the way down to the ear, and then begin a regular three-strand braid.

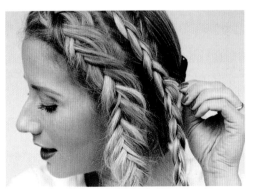

8. Spread out the braid for volume and tie it off with a clear elastic.

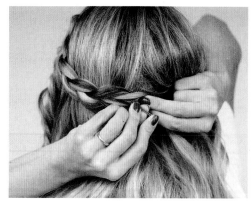

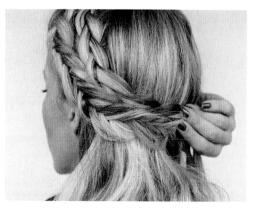

9. Pull the Dutch braid toward the opposite shoulder and secure around the crown with a bobby pin.

10. Drape the fishtail braid under the Dutch braid and secure with bobby pins.

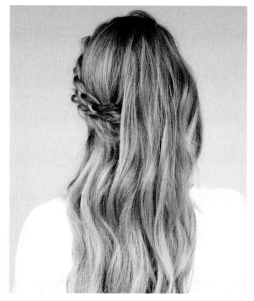

11. Remove the clip and let the rest of the hair fall over the pins.

Twist Me Pretty Braids

MIXED PONYTAIL

This is one of my favorite hairstyles to wear when my hair is dirty and I can't resurrect any curls!

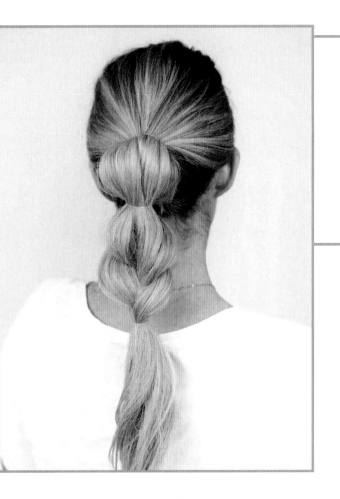

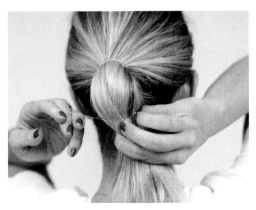

1. Pull the hair up into a ponytail and add a clear elastic a few inches down the tail.

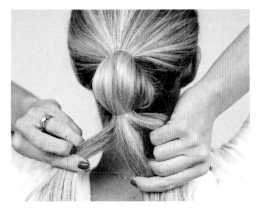

2. Split the tail below the elastic into three sections.

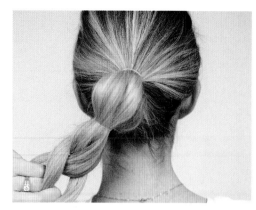

3. Braid a few inches down.

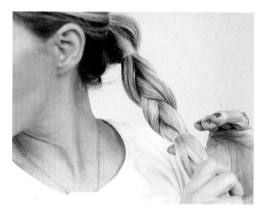

4. Secure the braid with a clear elastic.

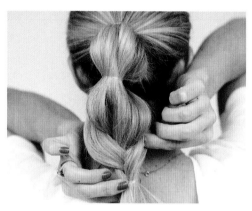

5. Tug and pull on the sections to make it look more full.

Twist Me Pretty Braids

PULL THROUGH PONYTAIL

This braid is super trendy right now! It's so versatile, and I love how the braid holds together, so if you have shorter layers or need a style that's not going to fall out, this is the one to choose!

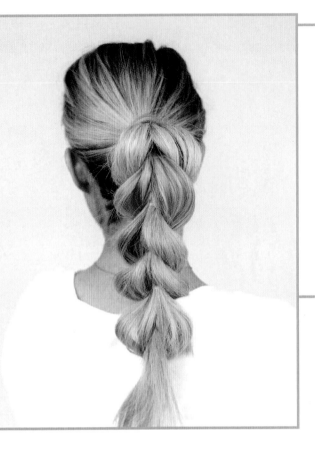

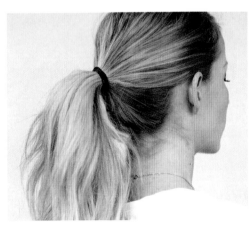

1. Pull the hair up into a ponytail.

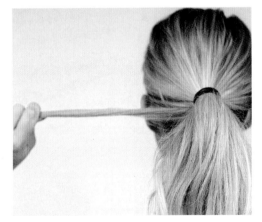

2. Take a small piece from underneath and wrap it around the elastic. Secure by wrapping a clear elastic around the section or by using a bobby pin.

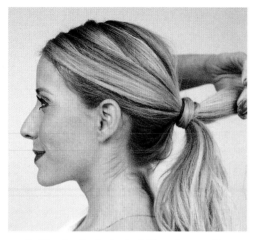

3. Split the hair in half horizontally.

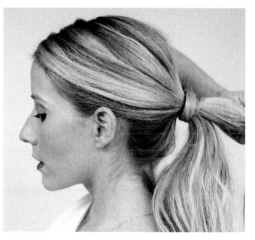

4. On the top section, add a clear elastic a couple inches down.

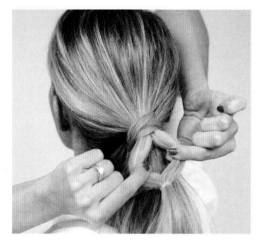

5. Create a hole in the center of the top section, right above the clear elastic.

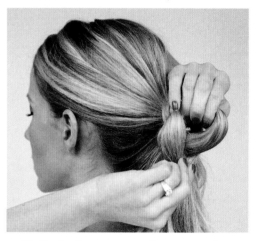

6. Pull the bottom section up and through.

Twist Me Pretty Braids

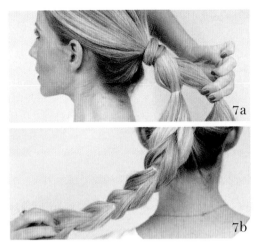

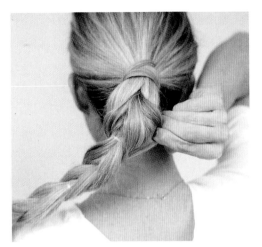

7a

7b

7. Now repeat those steps! Add another clear elastic a few inches down on the top strand, make a hole right above the elastic, and pull the bottom section through.

8. Now for my favorite part! Tug and pull on the sections to make the style look nice and chunky.

Pro Tip:

Use texturizing spray or styling mousse to help grip the sections and secure any flyaways!

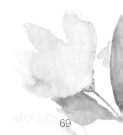

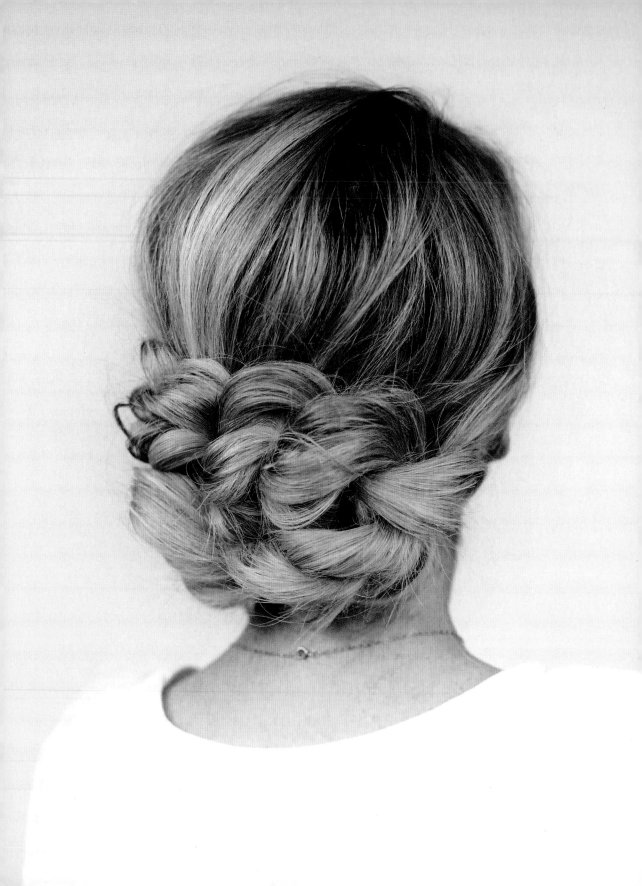

PULL THROUGH UPDO

This hairstyle works best on shorter hair but I wanted to include it because it's one of my most popular hairstyles. It's the perfect easy updo for those weddings and holiday parties!

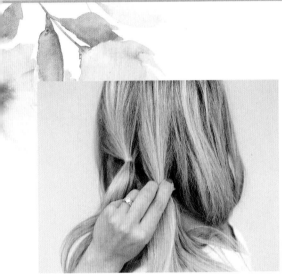

1. Put a small section of hair, right behind the ear, into a ponytail. Gather another section right next to it.

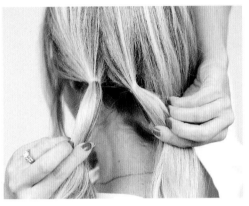

2. Secure the second section with a clear elastic so you have two ponytails side by side.

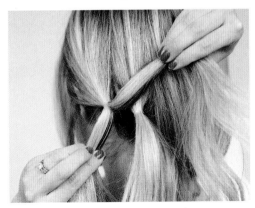

3. Split the first ponytail in two.

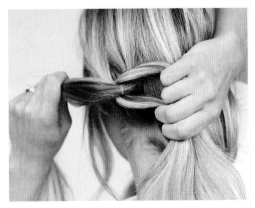

4. Wrap the sections of the first ponytail around the second ponytail.

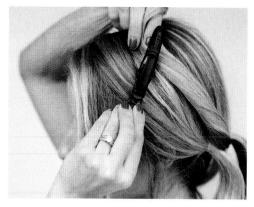

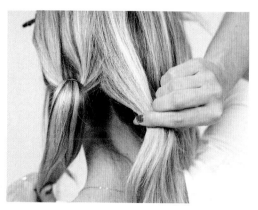

5. Secure the second ponytail's tail out of the way with a clip.

6. Holding the tails in one hand, use your other to gather a third section of hair. Combine the sections together and secure with a clear elastic.

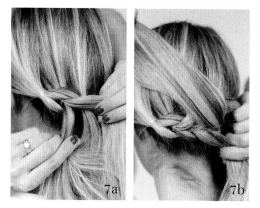

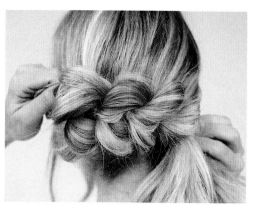

7. Remove the clip and repeat steps 3 through 6.

8. When you reach the other ear, tug and pull on the sections to make the braid look full.

Twist Me Pretty Braids

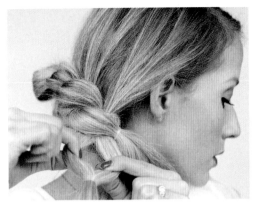

9. Add a clear elastic a couple inches down the bottom section. Create a hole in the center of that section.

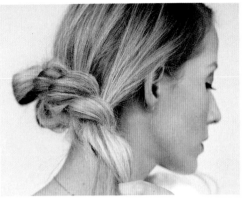

10. Pull the top section down and through the hole.

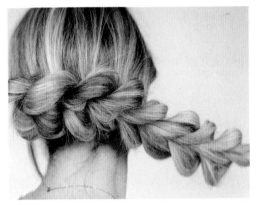

11. Continue your pull-through braid all the way down.

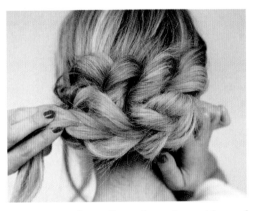

12. Wrap the tail to the other side and secure with bobby pins.

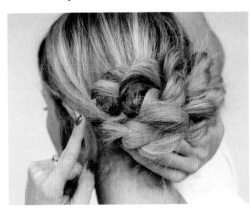

13. Tuck the tails into the bun and secure with bobby pins.

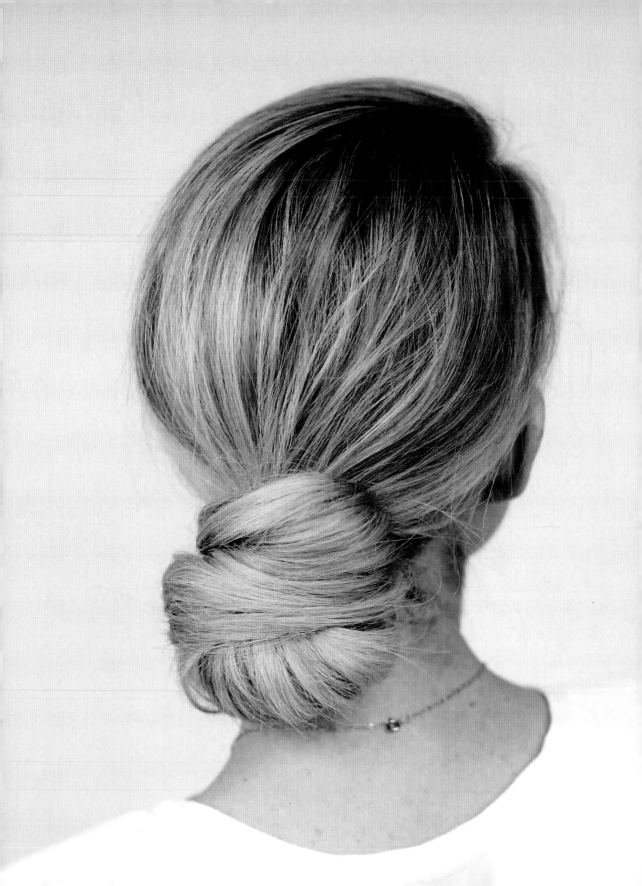

SIMPLE BUN

Proof that even the simplest of hairstyles can be some of the most beautiful!

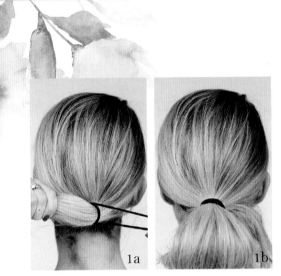

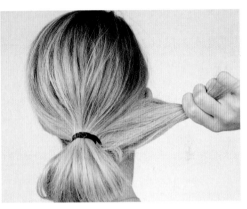

1. Pull the hair into a low bun, making sure to leave out enough ends to wrap around the top.

2. Gather the ends.

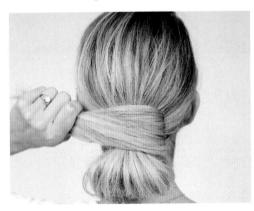

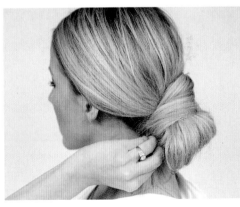

3. Wrap them over the top of the elastic.

4. Secure the ends underneath by threading them back through the elastic.

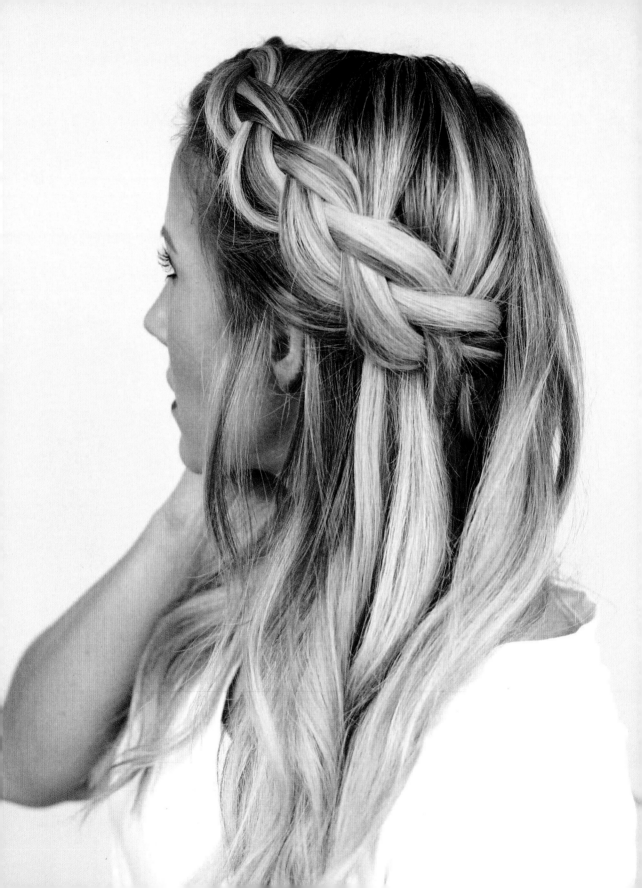

SOFT DUTCH BRAID

This is one of my favorite basic braids! I love how well it transitions from a day running errands to an elegant date night with my main squeeze. It's fast and easy, and the perfect style to build onto.

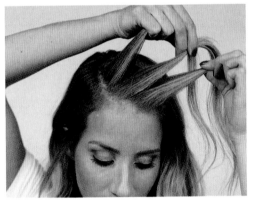

1. Gather a small section from the front and split it into three sections.

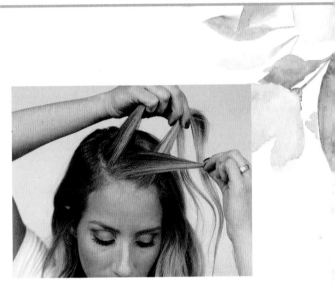

2. Braid the front section under the middle section.

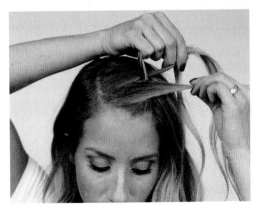

3. Braid the back section under the middle section.

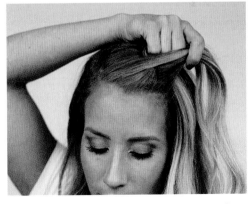

4. Add in a new section of hair to the front section.

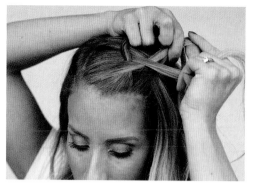

5. Braid it under the middle section.

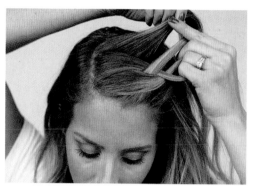

6. Add in a new section of hair to the back section and braid it under the middle section.

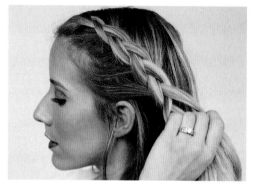

7. Continue Dutch braiding down to the ear.

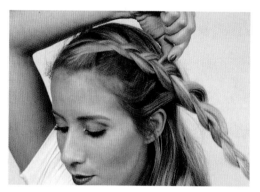

8. Finish with a regular three-strand braid all the way down to the ends. Gently tug on those sections to make the braid appear thicker.

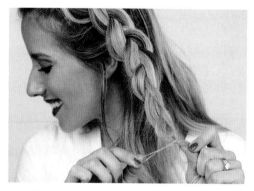

9. Tie off with a clear elastic.

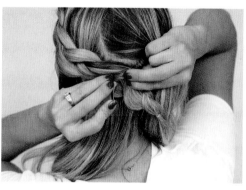

10. Drape the braid around the crown of the head, then secure with bobby pins. Sweep the hair that's down over the braid and let it fall over the pins.

SIDEWAYS DUTCH PONYTAIL

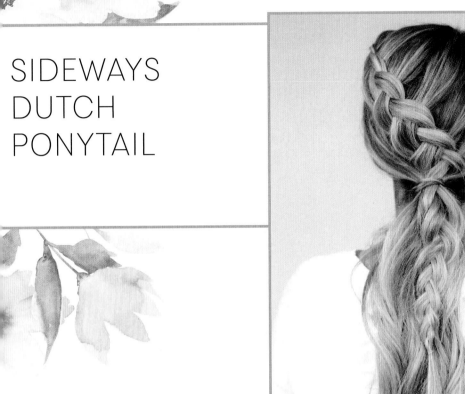

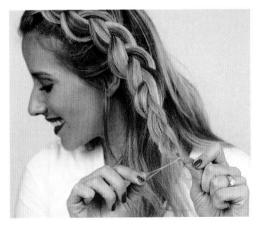

1. Start with the Soft Dutch Braid (page 77), but stop before step 10.

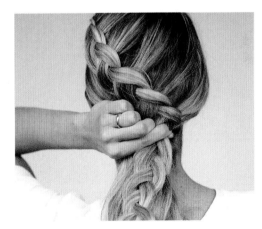

2. Gather all the hair and the braid.

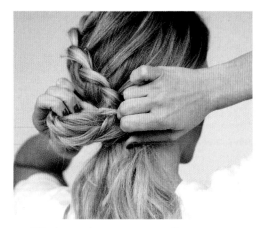

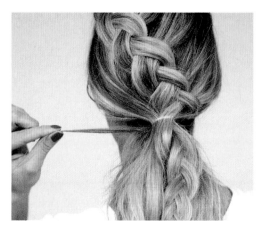

3. Tie it up into a ponytail.

4. Take a small section from underneath the ponytail and wrap it around the elastic, securing by either threading back through the elastic or pinning with a bobby pin.

TOPSY TAIL
HALF UP

You could leave this style as is, but there are many other ways to end it. You could continue the steps all the way down to create a beautiful braided look, or you could finish by tying the hair into a low messy bun. Remember to think outside the box!

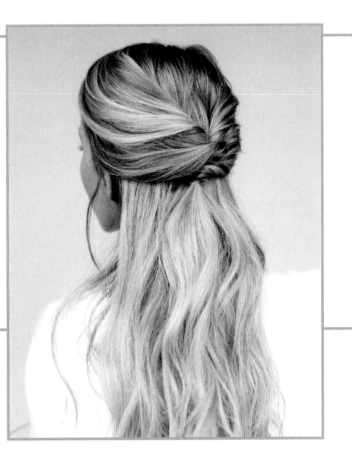

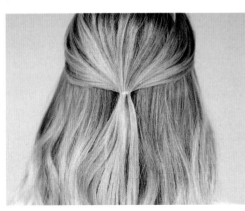

1. From the temples, pull the hair back into a half ponytail.

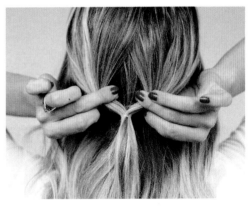

2. Split the hair right above the elastic.

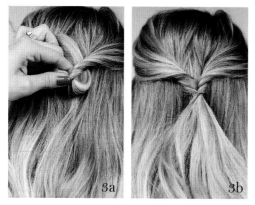

3. Flip the tail up and through the hole.

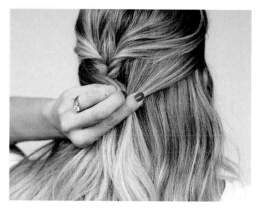

4. Gather two new sections, one from each side, and meet them just off center of the first topsy tail.

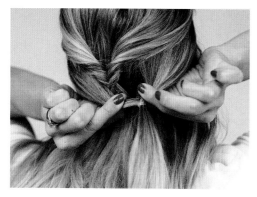

5. Secure with a clear elastic. Create a hole right above the elastic.

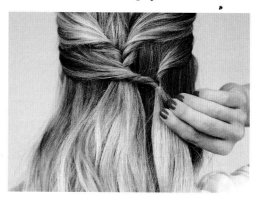

6. Flip the tail up and through the hole, creating your second topsy tail. This one should be just off center.

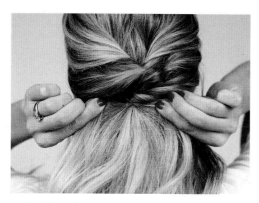

7. Make another topsy tail, only this time, create it on the opposite side of the one made in step 6.

Twist Me Pretty Braids

TRIPLE KNOTS

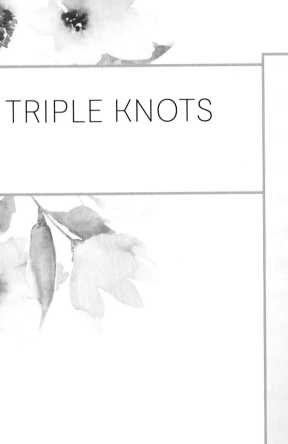

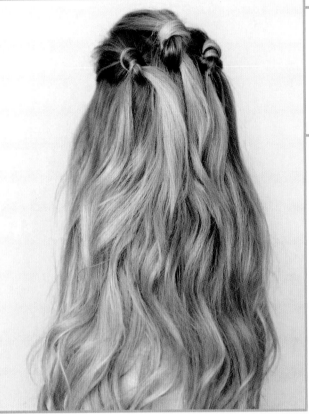

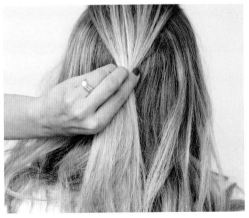

1. Pull back a small section of hair from the front of the head.

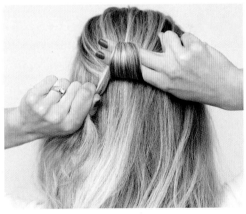

2. Place two fingers on top of the section and wrap the hair around them.

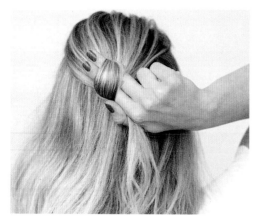

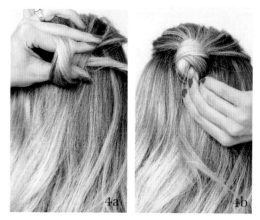

3. Hold the tail with your thumb.

4. With your other hand, reach through the loop and pull the tail through, creating your first knot.

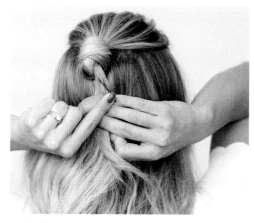

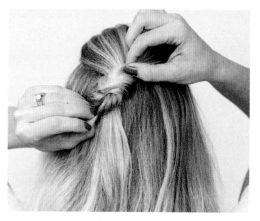

5. Take a bobby pin and secure the knot by threading it through the tail.

6. Tug on the knot to make it look more full and free.

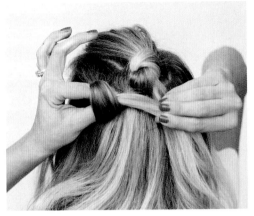

7. Gather another section of hair from the left side of your head, right near the temples. Repeat steps 1 through 6 on the left side of the head.

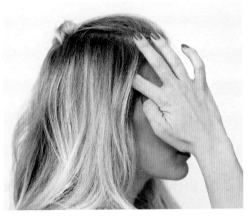

8. Gather another section of hair from the right side of your head, right near the temples.

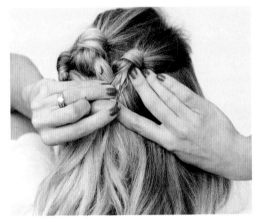

9. Create a third knot, following steps 1 through 6.

TWISTED CROWN BRAID

A very simple and elegant twist on your basic half-up style!

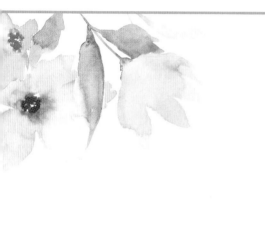

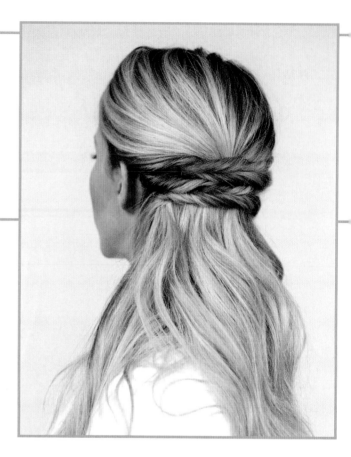

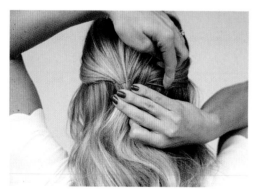

1. Pull the hair half up, and secure with crisscrossing bobby pins in the back.

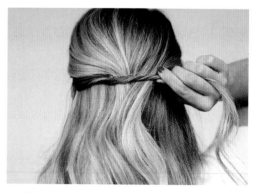

2. Take a small section from the front and twist it over the bobby pins.

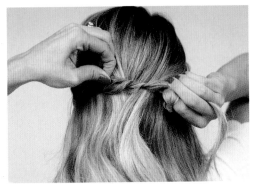

3. Loosen the twist by pulling it tight with one hand and tugging on the section with the other hand.

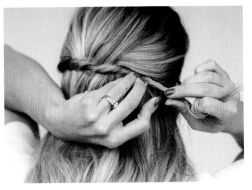

4. Secure the section with a bobby pin.

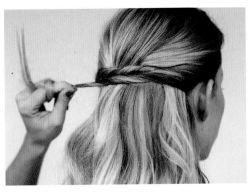

5. Take another small section from the front, on the opposite side, and drape it underneath the first twist. While pulling the whole twist tight with one hand, loosen it with the other hand.

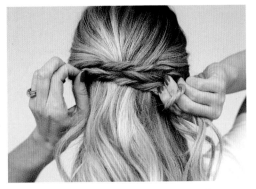

6. Repeat a few more times until you reach the bottom of your ears.

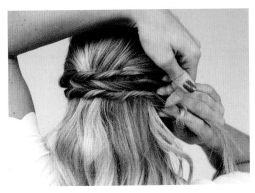

7. Secure the last section with a bobby pin.

TWISTED CROWN PONYTAIL

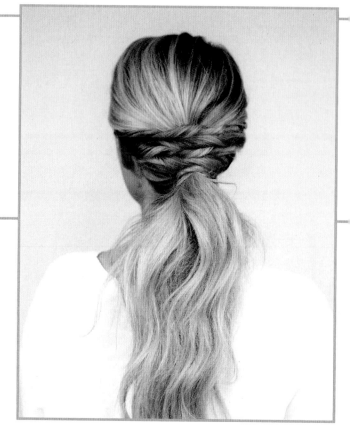

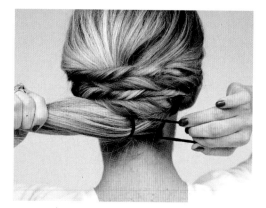

1. Start with the Twisted Crown Braid (page 86). Gather the remaining hair into a ponytail.

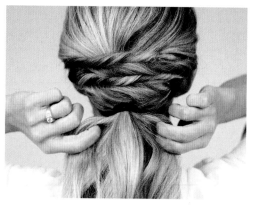

2. Cinch the ponytail by tugging the sides tight.

Twist Me Pretty Braids

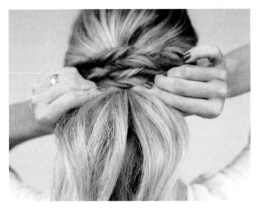

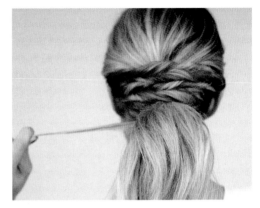

3. Cinch the sides tight enough that the ponytail falls right into the nape of the neck and underneath all the twists.

4. Take a small section from underneath and wrap it around the elastic.

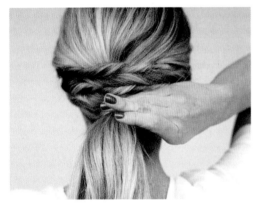

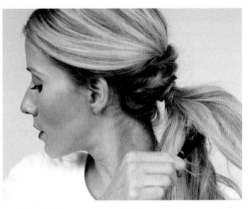

5. Secure it by threading it through the elastic, using a bobby pin, or my personal favorite, just adding a clear elastic over it.

6. Fluff the ponytail by teasing and adding texture.

Pro Tip:

Using dry shampoo or hairspray will give the ponytail a nice, full texture!

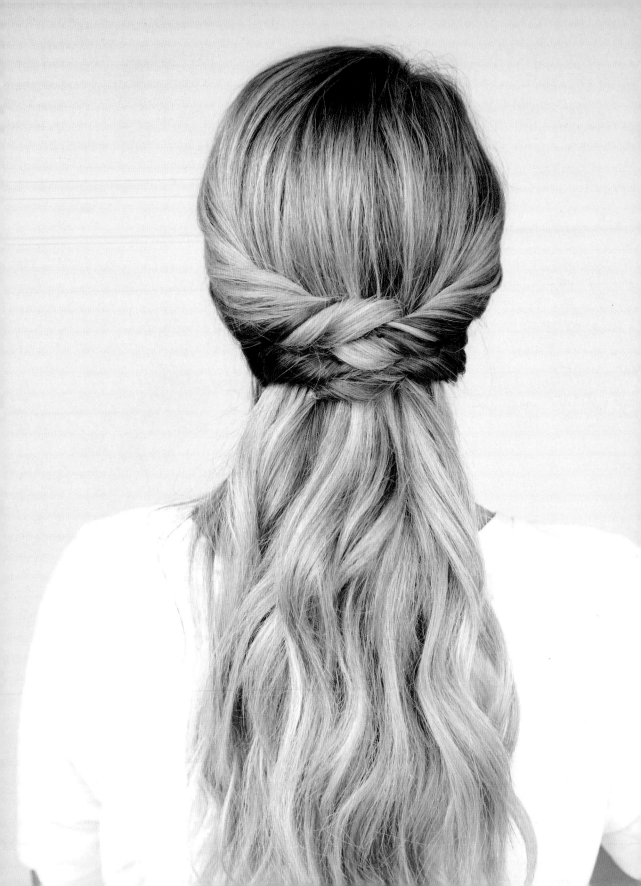

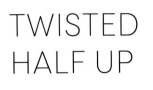

TWISTED HALF UP

This is one of my favorite half-up styles and I love it because it actually stays in place! I've seen a few hairstyles like this floating around that use bobby pins instead of clear elastics, but this technique keeps the hair from sliding down and the style from coming loose.

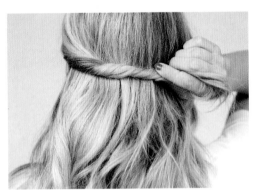

1. Pull a small section of hair from the left side of your head and twist it to the back.

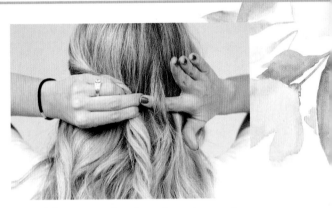

2. With your other hand, gather a tiny section of hair from the back of your head.

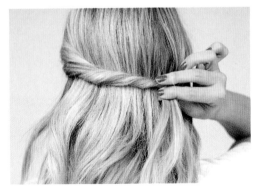

3. Tie the two sections together with a clear elastic.

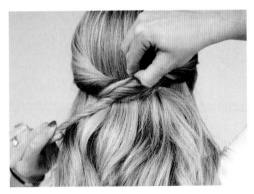

4. Pull another small section of hair from the front, this time from the right side, and twist it to the back. Go ahead and pull apart the twist to make it look a little more undone and full.

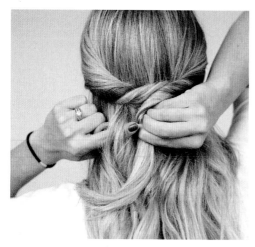

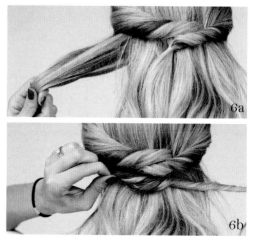

5. Gather a tiny section of hair with your other hand, right below the first twist, and secure the second twist to this new section with a clear elastic.

6. Twist back another section of hair from the front, right below the first section, and secure it to a smaller section on the opposite side.

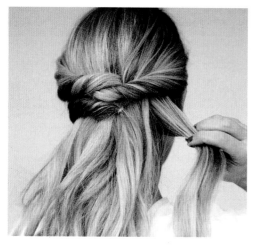

7. Repeat until you have two sections pulled back from each side.

Twist Me Pretty Braids

TWISTED HALF PONYTAIL

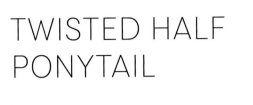

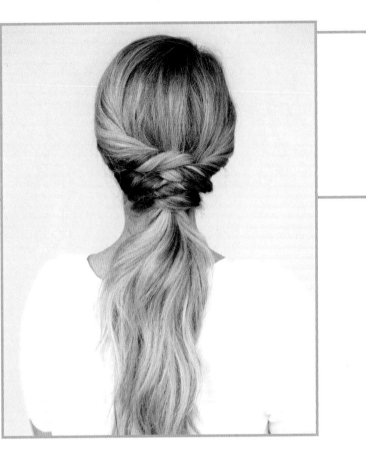

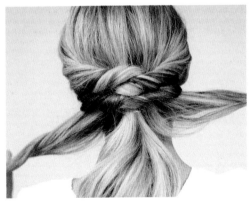

1. Start with the Twisted Half Up hairstyle (page 91). Divide the remaining hair into three sections.

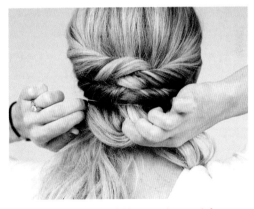

2. Secure the middle section with a clear elastic.

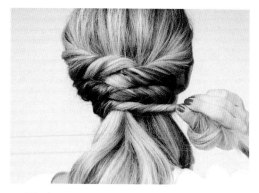

3. Twist one section over the ponytail.

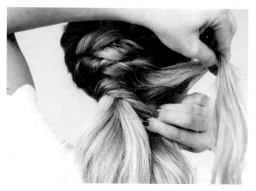

4. While holding the twist in place, gather the other section of hair with your opposite hand.

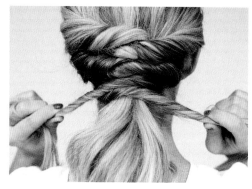

5. Twist it and wrap it around the ponytail.

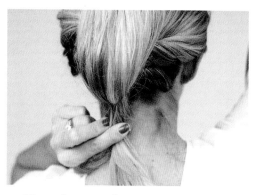

6. Now that you have two crossed twists, wrap them underneath the ponytail and hold them in place with your thumb and index finger.

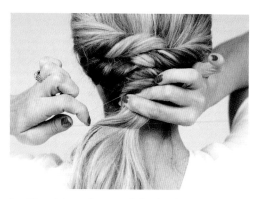

7. Combine them with the larger ponytail and secure by wrapping a clear elastic around the entire ponytail.

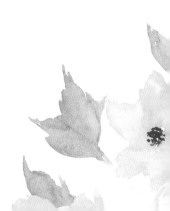

Twist Me Pretty Braids

TWISTED
CROWN

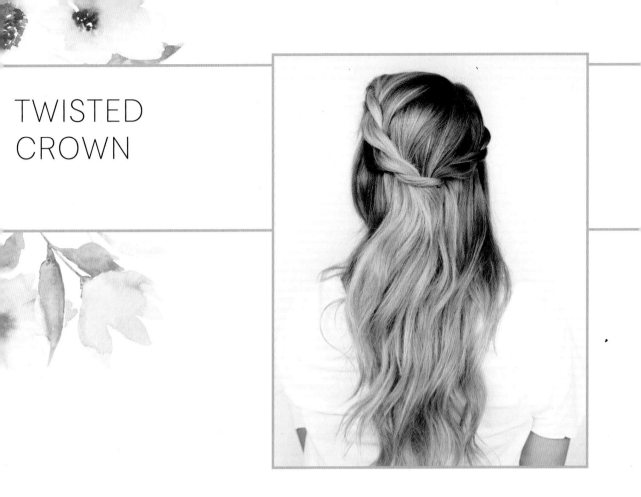

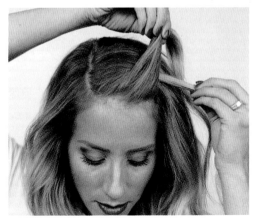

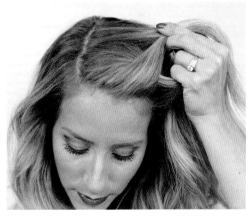

1. Gather a small section of hair from the front, on the heavier side of your part. Split it in two sections, and twist the front section over the back section.

2. Add a new section of hair to the back section.

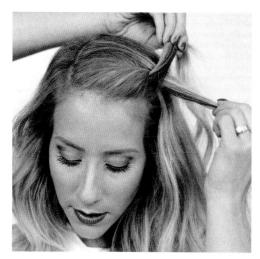

3. Add a new section of hair to the front section and then twist it over the back section.

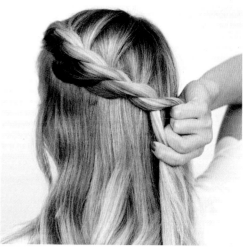

4. Continue twisting and adding in new sections of hair on each side until you reach the back of your head.

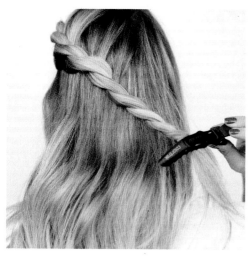

5. Finish with a regular twist all the way down and secure with a clip or elastic.

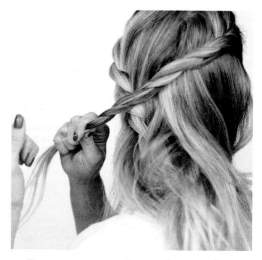

6. Repeat steps 1 through 5 on the other side.

Twist Me Pretty Braids

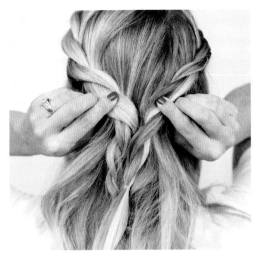

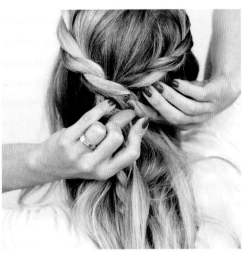

7. Pull the twists together at the crown and fold one twist over the other.

8. Secure the twists with a bobby pin and remove the elastic or clip from the bottom of the twists.

Pro Tip:

When bobby pinning, you only need to secure the very front section of a larger piece of hair. That front section will hold the rest of hair in place!

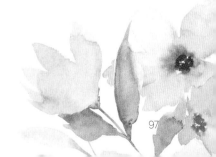

TWISTED PONYTAIL

Another favorite, this hairstyle lends itself to many other styles. You could put the ends into a fishtail braid or you could tie it up into a messy bun or elegant updo.

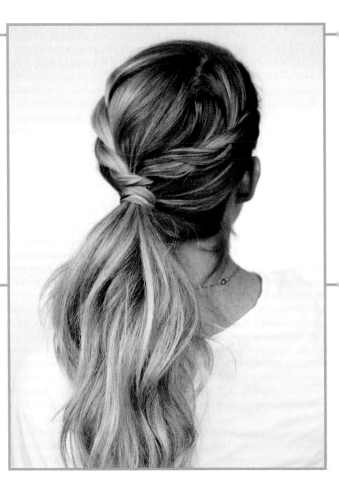

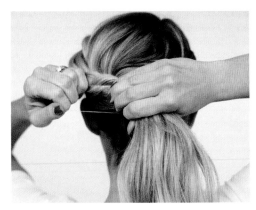

1. Style your hair in a Twisted Crown (page 95). Pull the remaining hair into a ponytail.

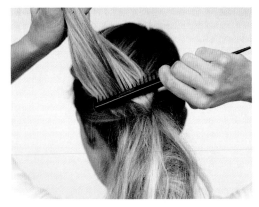

2. Tease the tail with a comb.

Twist Me Pretty Braids

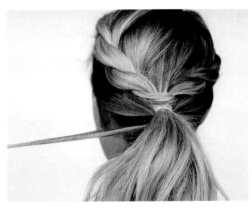

3. Gather a small section of hair from underneath.

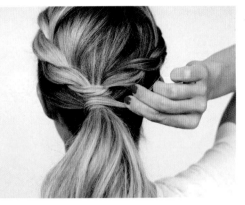

4. Wrap it around the clear elastic.

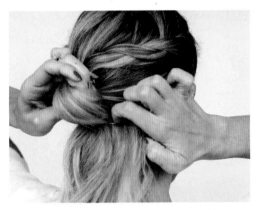

5. Secure the piece of hair by adding another clear elastic on top.

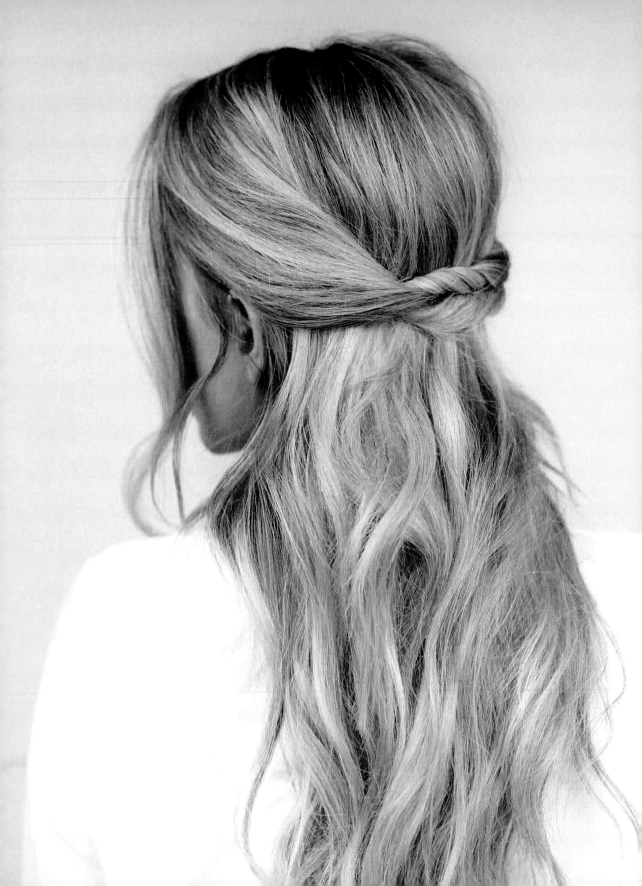

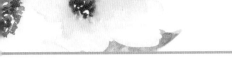

TWISTED TOGETHER

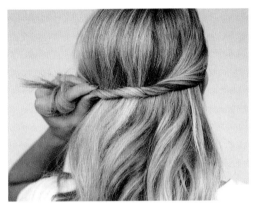

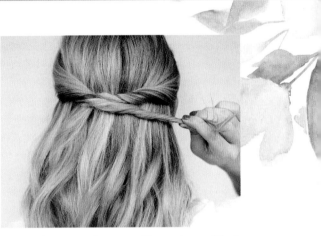

1. Gather a small section of hair from one side of the head, twist it across the crown, and bobby pin it in place.

2. Gather another small section of hair from the other side of the head, then twist it across the crown, tucking the tail slightly under the first twist.

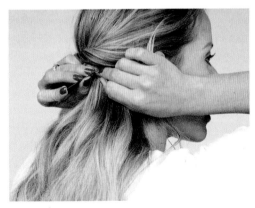

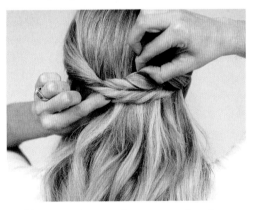

3. Bobby pin the tail in place. Remember, you only need to snag a tiny section in front of the twist with the bobby pin to hold the entire twist in place.

4. Tug on the sections to make the twists seem more full and voluminous.

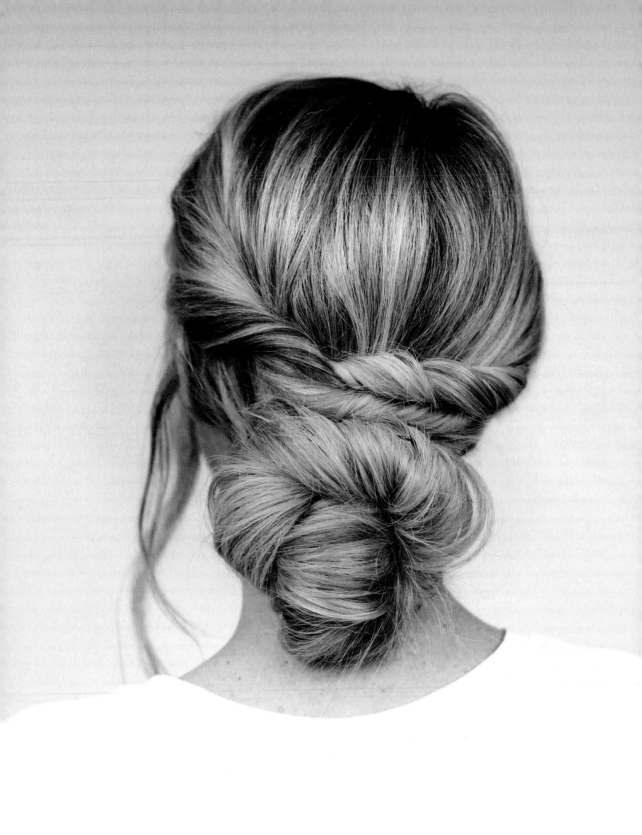

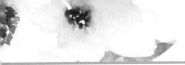

TWISTED
TOGETHER BUN

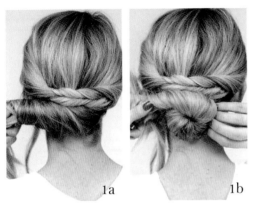

1a   1b

1. Create the Twisted Together style (page 101). Roll the remaining hair into a ballerina bun.

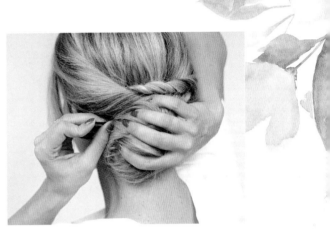

2. Secure the bun with bobby pins as you go.

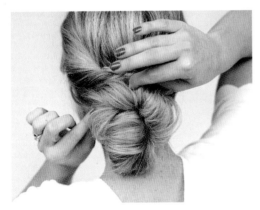

3. Pull apart the bun to make it look a little more undone, or finish with a strong-hold hairspray to keep that sleek elegant bun look.

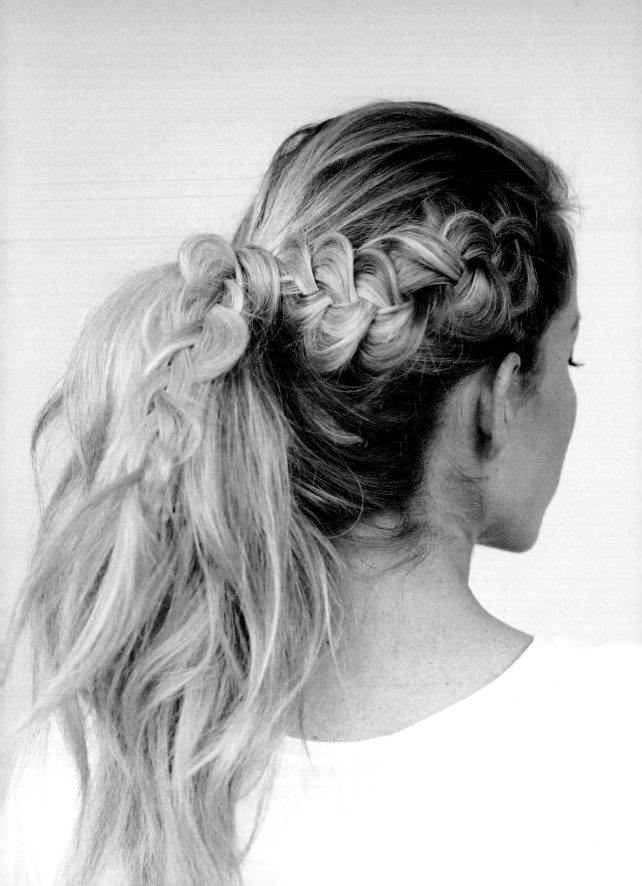

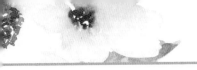

VIKING BRAID

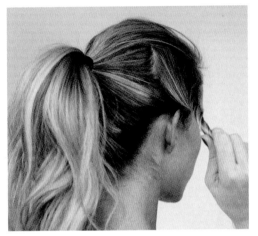

1. Pull the hair up into a ponytail, leaving out a small section of hair right above the ear.

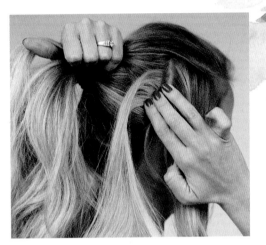

2. If needed, clip in a single weft extension right behind the section left out of the ponytail.

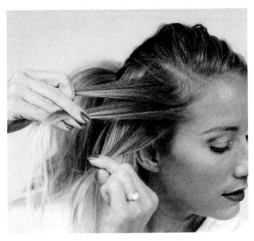

3. Divide the section into three.

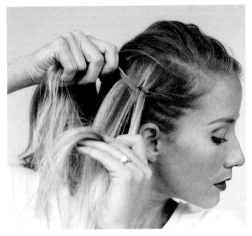

4. Begin Dutch braiding the hair back.

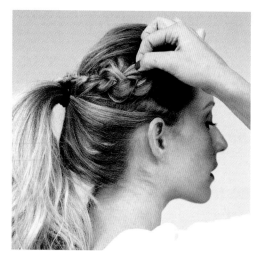

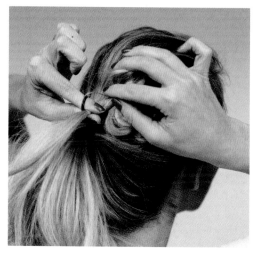

5. When you get to the end, pull apart and tug on those sections to make the braid look bigger.

6. Thread the braid into the elastic holding the ponytail in place.

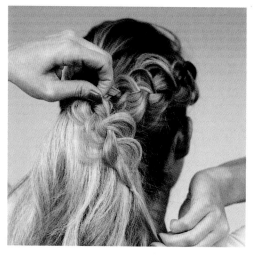

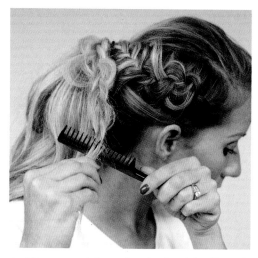

7. Continue pulling apart and tugging on those pieces to give dimension to the braid.

8. You can either tie the braid off with a clear elastic, or tease the ends and spray well with hairspray. The snarls will hold the braid in place.

Twist Me Pretty Braids

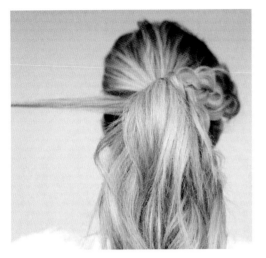

Pro Tip:

Using single weft extensions in your braids is an easy way to add thickness and dimension, and they're easy to hide when the braid is fluffed out. Don't let the big braids on Instagram fool you; they're almost always styled with extensions!

9. Take a small section from underneath the ponytail and wrap it around the elastic. Either thread the hair through the original ponytail, or add a new clear elastic on top to secure the strand.

UNEVEN CENTER BRAID

I'm just a tiny bit obsessed with this braid! It's super quick to style and so undone and effortless looking. It also has great texture and shows all the different colors in the hair!

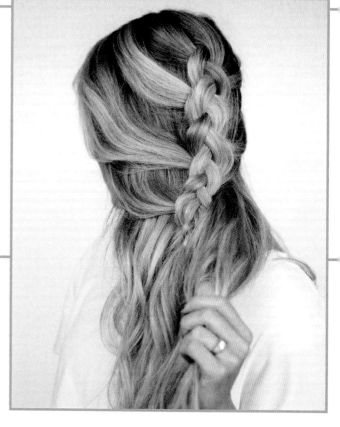

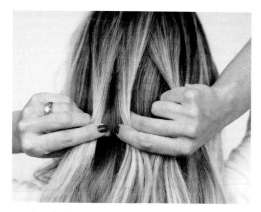

1. Gather a small section of hair from the back and split it into three.

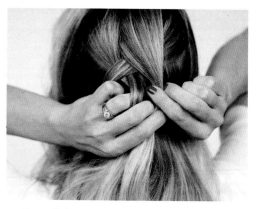

2. Dutch braid one stitch.

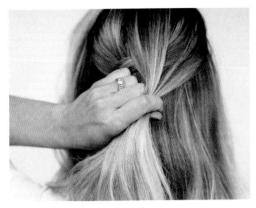

3. Add in a new section of hair to one side.

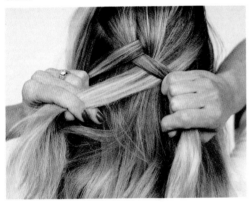

4. Braid it under the middle section.

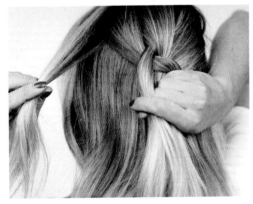

5. Add in a new section of hair to the other side.

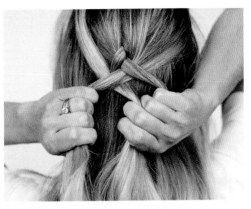

6. Braid it under the middle section.

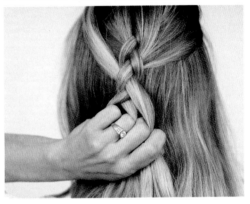

7. Braid the hair one stitch without adding in any new sections of hair.

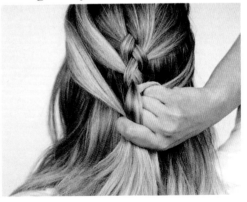

8. Add in a new section of hair to one side. Braid it under the middle. Add in a new section of hair to the other side, then braid it under the middle.

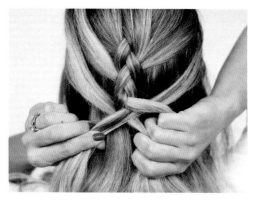

9. Repeat these steps by alternating when you add in new sections of hair and when you don't.

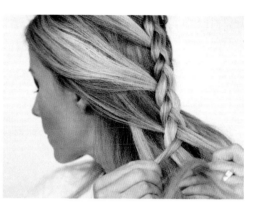

10. When you get several stitches down, finish the braid off with a regular three-strand braid.

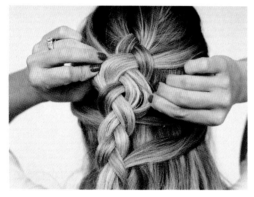

11. Pull apart the braid to make it look more full and undone.

Pro Tip:

Style this braid on second-day hair so the sections will hold better and it'll have a nicer texture to play with. If you need, spray some dry shampoo into the roots to absorb any unwanted oils.

Twist Me Pretty Braids

FOUR-STRAND BRAID

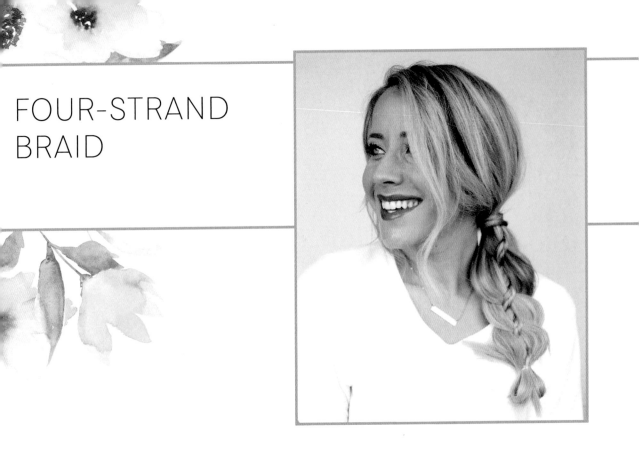

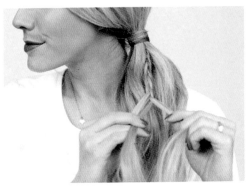

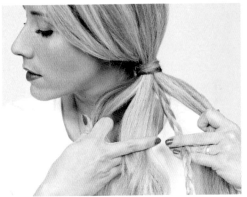

1. Pull the hair over into a side ponytail. Optionally, you can wrap a small piece of hair around the elastic and secure with a bobby pin or add a new clear elastic over the ponytail.

Take a long layer from the ponytail and braid a simple three-strand braid all the way down, then secure with a clear elastic.

2. Divide the rest of the ponytail into three sections. You should now have four sections, including the braid. The strand closest to the face is #1, then comes #2, the braided strand is #3, and #4 is farthest from your face.

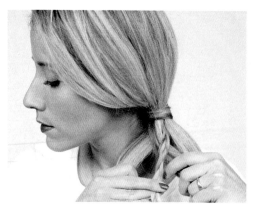

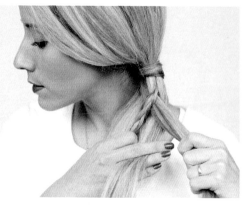

3. Take strand #1 over strand #2 and then take the braid over strand #2.

4. Take strand #4 under strand #3.

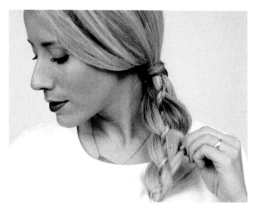

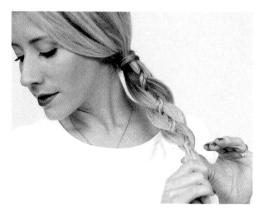

5. Take strand #3 under strand #4. Then repeat steps 3 through 5 until you reach the ends.

7. Gently tug on the sections to make the braid look bigger.

6. Tie off with a clear elastic.

Pro Tip:

If I cross an outer section over the middle, then I'm going to take the braid over the middle. If I'm crossing an outer section under the middle, then I'm going to take the braid under the middle. The braided strand shouldn't be moving around a whole lot; it should be staying in the center!

If you are struggling with this hairstyle, make sure to find me on YouTube so you can see every step in action!!

DRAPED WATERFALL BRAID

This is one of my absolute favorite hairstyles. The steps are a little tedious, but once you get the hang of it, it's actually a very easy braid! This is also a great braid to mix with other hairstyles! If you are struggling following along with any of these step-by-steps, check out my YouTube channel and watch the video tutorials!

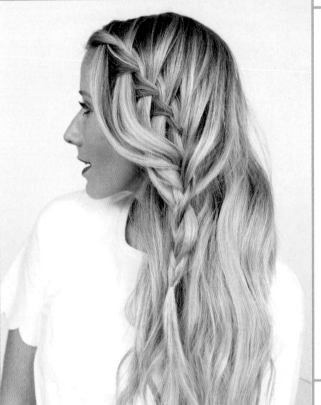

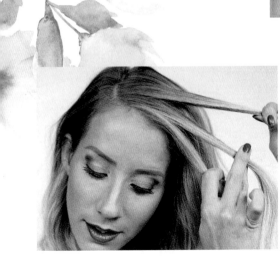

1. Give the hair a side part and split a small section into three.

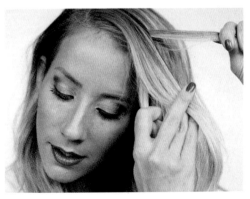

2. Take the top strand over the middle section.

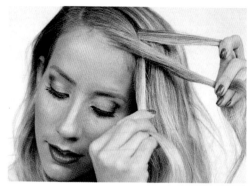

3. Take the bottom strand over the middle section.

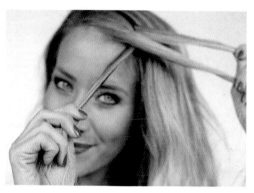

4. Grab the bottom section, the section that's hanging down, and bring it forward.

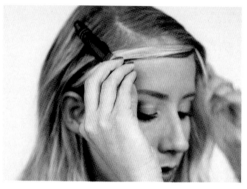

5. Clip it out of the way on the other side.

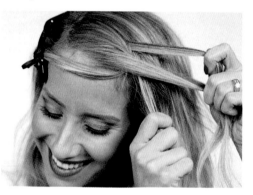

6. Gather a new section of hair to replace the one you sectioned off.

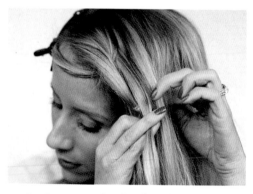

7. And now we're back to having three strands!

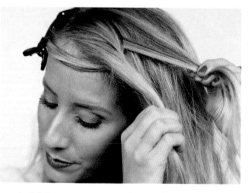

8. Add in a new section of hair to the top strand.

Twist Me Pretty Braids

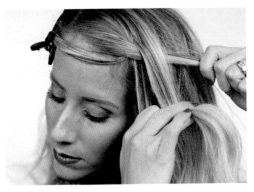

9. Braid the top strand over the middle section.

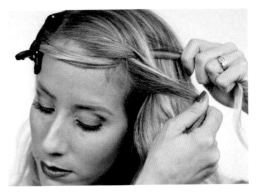

10. Braid the bottom strand over the middle section. Then repeat steps 4 through 10.

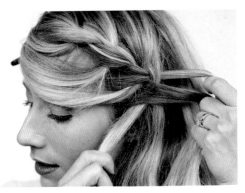

11. Keep repeating steps 4 through 10 until you have about five sections pulled to the other side!

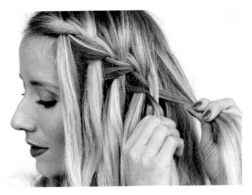

12. When you get to your ear, remove the clip, and let the sections fall. Add a new section of hair to the top strand and braid it over the middle.

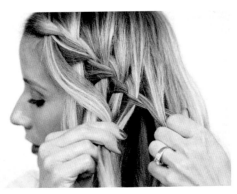

13. Add the first waterfall section to the bottom strand and braid it over the middle. Then add in a new section of hair to the top strand and braid it over the middle.

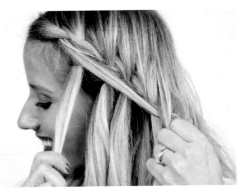

14. Add in the second waterfall section to the bottom strand and braid it over the middle.

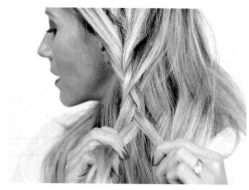

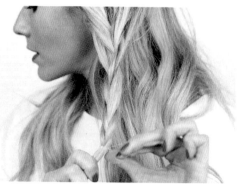

15. Once all the sections of the waterfall are added back into the braid, finish the style off by doing a regular three-strand braid all the way to the ends.

16. Secure with a clear elastic.

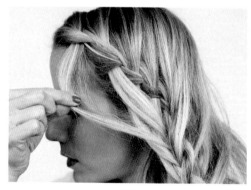

Did you do it? Does it look amazing?! I'm tellin' ya, it's one of my favorite mixed braids ever! If you're still struggling, make sure to watch the video. It'll give you clarity on all those blank spaces!

17. Loosen the waterfall sections up just a bit so that the style lays nicely and you can see all the detail in the braid!

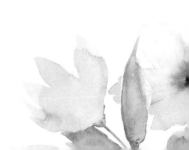

Twist Me Pretty Braids

DRAPED WATERFALL FISHTAIL BRAID

The Draped Waterfall Braid is one of my favorite buildable hairstyles. You can basically attach any braid or bun to it, as done here with the fishtail braid, and it gives the style just a little bit more interest and character!

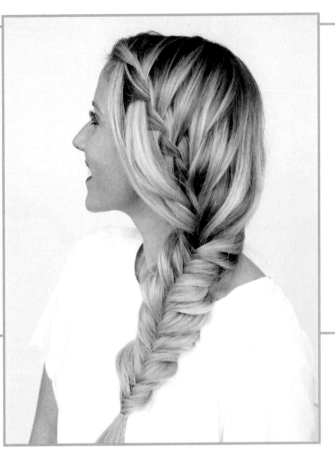

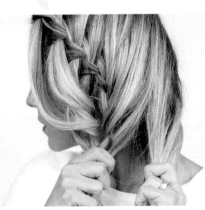

1. Start with the Draped Waterfall Braid (page 113).

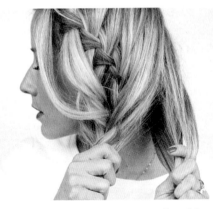

2. Pull the hair over to one shoulder, then split it into two equal sections.

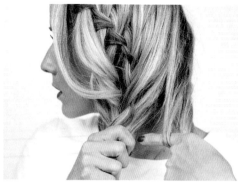

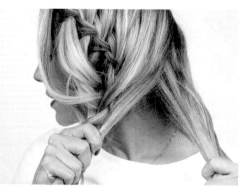

3. Holding one section with each hand, knuckles forward, use your index finger to take a small sliver of hair from the back section.

4. Grab that sliver with your other hand and combine it with the front section.

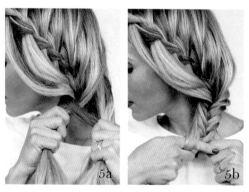

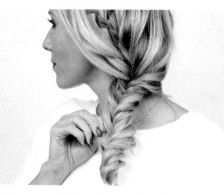

5. Repeat on the other side and continue braiding down until your fishtail braid starts forming. Keep your sections tight and small!

6. Secure with a clear elastic and pull on the fishtail braid to make it look more full and voluminous.

Pro Tip:

The smaller the sections, the more detailed the braid. If you want a super-fluffy fishtail braid, try passing larger sections back and forth! Also, really focus on just rotating your wrist when passing the sections. I've found it really helps me to keep the braid clean and the steps organized!

Twist Me Pretty Braids

WATERFALL MESSY BUN

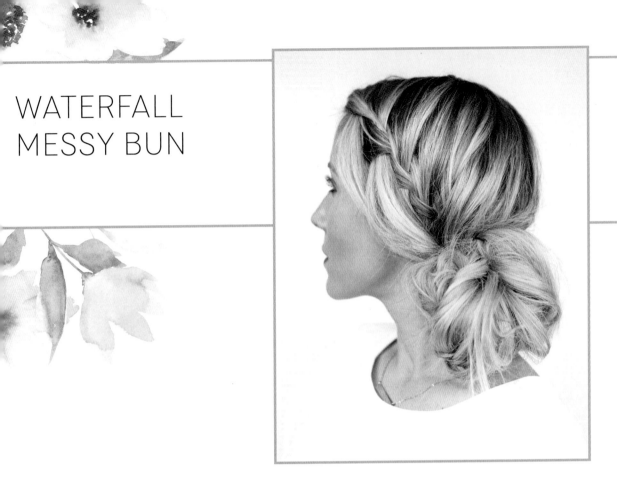

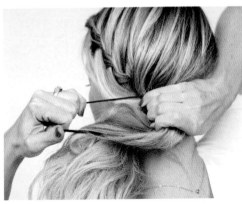

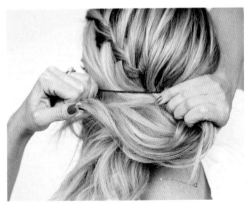

1. Start by creating the Draped Waterfall Braid hairstyle (page 113). Pull the hair through an elastic. Make sure it's off center and right below the braid.

2. Continue pulling the hair through the elastic.

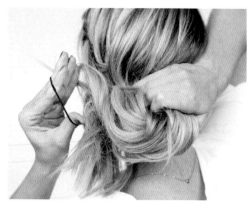

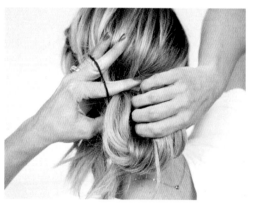

3. Make sure to twist the elastic right before the ends fall out of the ponytail.

4. Cover the bun with the hand that has the elastic on it.

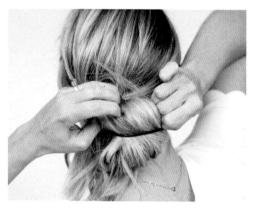

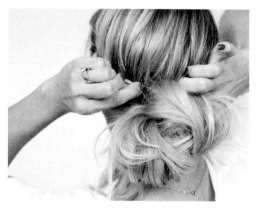

5. Pull the elastic over the bun.

6. Finish it off by cinching up on the bun to make it more tight, and secure where you want with bobby pins.

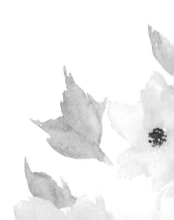

Twist Me Pretty Braids

CORSET BRAID

This is such a fun and unique braid! It's a waterfall braid on one side and then a French braid on the other. The twist is that we incorporate the dropped sections from our waterfall braid into our French braid! Let's get to it, shall we?!

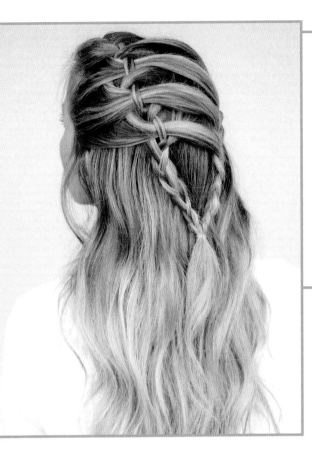

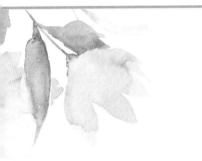

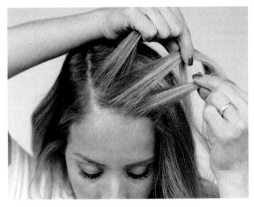

1. Take a section from the front, on the heavier side of your part, and divide it into three sections.

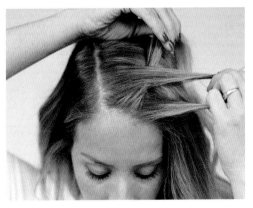

2. Braid the top strand over the middle section.

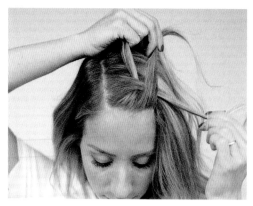

3. Braid the bottom strand over the middle section.

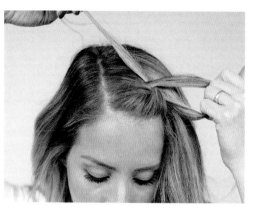

4. Take that middle strand under the top strand.

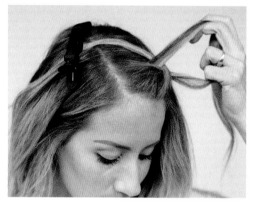

5. Secure the middle strand on the other side with a clip.

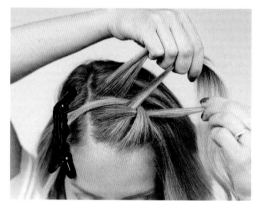

6. Replace the clipped strand with a new section of hair.

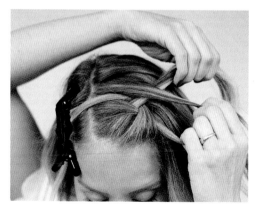

7. Cross that new section over the middle.

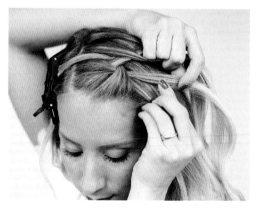

8. Add in more hair to the bottom section.

Twist Me Pretty Braids

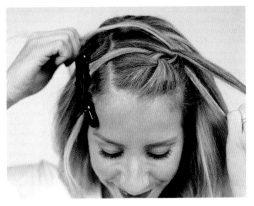

9. Braid it over the middle, and then take it under the top strand.

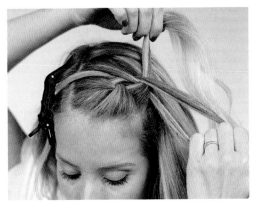

10. Secure the middle strand on the other side with a clip.

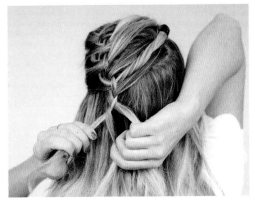

11. Continue your waterfall braid until you reach the back of your head.

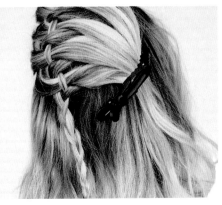

12. Continue braiding all the way to the ends, and then tie the braid off with a clear elastic.

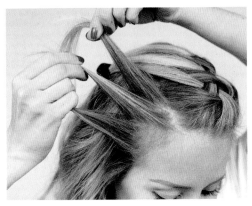

13. Gather a section from the other side of your head, and split it into three equal parts.

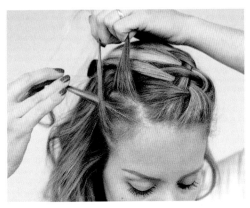

14. Braid the bottom strand over the middle.

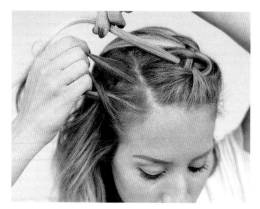

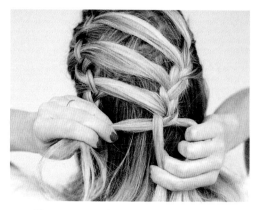

15. Add in the first clipped section from your waterfall braid to the top strand and then braid it over the middle.

16. Repeat until you run out of sections to add in, finish with a three-strand braid, and then secure the braids together with a clear elastic.

Twist Me Pretty Braids

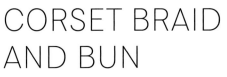

CORSET BRAID AND BUN

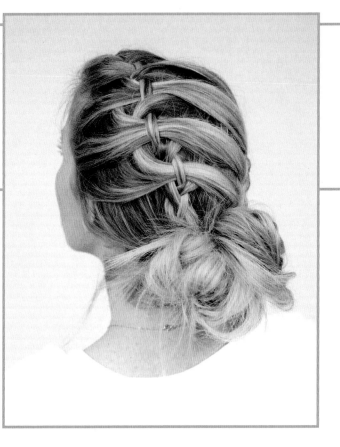

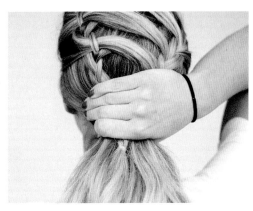

1. Start with the Corset Braid (page 121). Gather the hair into a ponytail.

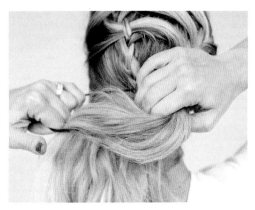

2. Pull the hair through an elastic.

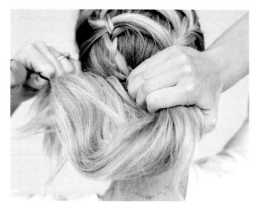

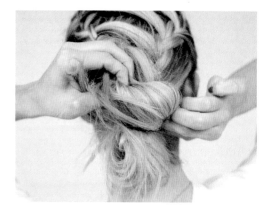

3. Make sure to twist the elastic right before the ends fall out of the ponytail.

4. Cover the bun with the hand that has the elastic on it and pull the elastic over the bun with your other hand.

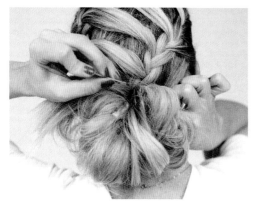

5. Finish it off by cinching up on the bun to make it more tight, and secure where you want with bobby pins.

About the Author

Abby Smith is a stay-at-home mom to 4 young children, a content creator, and online influencer. She has been blogging since 2011 and has created a community of women who share her values and passion for life.

She started her YouTube channel in 2014 and has gained over 300K subscribers who tune in to her weekly tutorials and vlogs.

Abby is a full-blown optimist, goal digger, successful author, and entrepreneur. She is a skilled photographer, videographer, and believes the quote from Thomas Monson that you don't find the happy life, you make it.

Find more of Abby's work at twistmepretty.com.

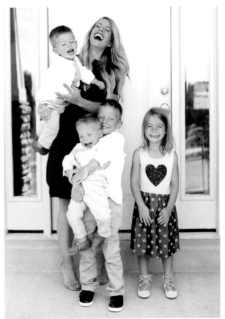

Brian Smith